Dennis B. Worthen, PhD

Pharmacy in World War II

Pre-publication REVIEWS, COMMENTARIES, EVALUATIONS . . .

"**D**rug product and manpower shortages; emergency preparedness; questions about adequate numbers of faculty and the length and essential elements of a pharmacy curriculum; the need to strengthen state pharmacy practice acts. A snapshot of pharmacy's past or a description of contemporary issues in pharmacy? Dennis Worthen has captured the critical elements of our professional roots and those 'evergreen' issues we still struggle with today. Notably, this book also reveals the strategic nature of the mid-twentieth century, when extraordinarily important advances were made by strong leaders in our profession. Accreditation of pharmacy schools, formation of the American Foundation for Pharmaceutical Education, creation of a model pharmacy practice act, and the expansion in numbers of women entering pharmacy education and practice are the building blocks of quality upon which our profession stands firm today."

Lucinda L. Maine, PhD
Executive Vice President,
American Association of Colleges
of Pharmacy

"**T**his is a well-researched book on the events and circumstances that not only shaped pharmacy during World War II, but the future of the profession as well. Dr. Worthen's research on this important era demonstrates his passion for pharmacy and fills a void in our history. This is a must-read for historians, service men and women, and those interested in understanding workforce issues. This would have been an invaluable resource during my tenure as a pharmacy manpower analyst for the Bureau of Health Professions.

The book chronicles the struggles and determination of the leadership of APhA to gain recognition of the pharmacist as a health care provider in the services, and ultimately the creation of the Pharmacy Corps. It also provides important insights into the contributions to the war effort by drugstores. Individual stories add a special touch to varied pharmacist roles during World War II."

Fred G. Paavola, RPh, DSc, FAPhA
Rear Admiral, USPHS Retired;
Chief of Staff, AZ-1 DMAT

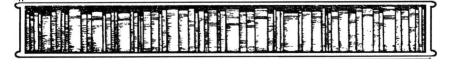

More pre-publication
REVIEWS, COMMENTARIES, EVALUATIONS . . .

"Dr. Worthen's love of pharmacy and passion for telling the story of how pharmacists contributed to the United State's victory in World War II, permeate the pages of this extraordinary book, a tour de force of research, project management, and writing. Contemporary pharmacists reading this book will discover that many of the hot issues of today were also vexing the profession's leaders in the early 1940s: the public image of pharmacists, appropriate use of pharmacist's talents, pharmacist shortages, the role of pharmacy technicians, and the role of pharmacies in emergency preparedness and homeland security. Especially valuable is the history of organized pharmacy's efforts to persuade the military to recognize pharmacy practice as a professional service that is essential for the safe use of medicines and to accord pharmacists commensurate status as officers. This book is an important, lively addition to the record of pharmacy's service to the public and the national interest."

William A. Zellmer, MPH
Deputy Executive Vice President,
American Society of Health-System
Pharmacists

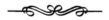

"There are hundreds of books capturing various aspects of World War II, but this is the very first devoted to pharmacy. Dennis Worthen engagingly critiques the economic, educational, organizational, and societal factors influencing pharmacy on both the home front and in the military. The author also contributes one of the first published accounts of the role of pharmacy in the U.S. military from the Revolutionary War to the creation of the U.S. Pharmacy Corps in 1943 and the 1947 establishment of the Medical Service Corps. World War II veterans, as well as WWII history buffs, will especially appreciate the memories recorded by those who survived combat action. They include a hospital pharmacist who was in Honolulu when the Japanese attacked; a Navy officer whose ship was sunk at Slapton Sands in England; several Coast Guardsmen who landed troops in their LSTs at Normandy and Salerno; an infantryman in the Battle of the Bulge; a Marine who landed on Iwo Jima; and an Army infantryman who invaded New Guinea."

George B. Griffenhagen, MS
Pharmacist; WWII Veteran;
Former Editor, *Journal of the*
American Pharmaceutical Association

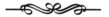

"The voices of American pharmacy's 'greatest generation' speak to us in Dennis Worthen's new book *Pharmacy in World War II*. The author has filled a gap in the historical literature and placed this critical period for pharmacy in the broader context of the era. Readers will come away with a better understanding of both pharmacy and American society in the 1940s. After describing pharmacy's general failure to get appropriate consideration from the Selective Service, Worthen provides the definitive story of the profession's pursuit of a Pharmacy Corps within the Army. He also adds extensive documentation and appendixes rich in data. *Pharmacy in World War II* is an important book for a profession now at another crossroads. Worthen shows how American pharmacy coped with the nation's greatest crisis and came through revived and ready for new challenges. The historical lessons contained in this work should inspire pharmacy's leaders of today and tomorrow."

Gregory J. Higby, PhD, RPh
Director, American Institute
of the History of Pharmacy

More pre-publication
REVIEWS, COMMENTARIES, EVALUATIONS . . .

"**D**r. Worthen has done an incredible job in putting this book together; it is difficult to put it down once you start reading. The book is filled with information and data that is informative, even shocking at times. The establishment of the 'Memories Project Files' will serve pharmacy historians for years into the future. The information contained in the book, including the epilogue, is fascinating. I learned a great deal about pharmacy, pharmacists, WWII, and the sacrifices that were made as well as the maturation of the profession during those years. Dr. Worthen has done pharmacy a unique and valuable service in documenting our profession during this critical period of our nation's history; a time that allowed us to remain a free nation and to practice our honored profession."

Loyd V. Allen, Jr., PhD, RPh
Professor Emeritus, University of Oklahoma College of Pharmacy; Editor-in-Chief, *International Journal of Pharmaceutical Compounding*

Pharmaceutical Products Press®
An Imprint of The Haworth Press, Inc.
New York • London • Oxford

Pharmacy
in World War II

PHARMACEUTICAL PRODUCTS PRESS
Pharmaceutical Heritage:
Pharmaceutical Care Through History
Mickey C. Smith, PhD
Dennis B. Worthen, PhD
Senior Editors

Laboratory on the Nile: A History of the Wellcome Tropical Research Laboratories by Patrick F. D'Arcy

America's Botanico-Medical Movements: Vox Populi by Alex Berman and Michael A. Flannery

Medicines for the Union Army: The United States Army Laboratories During the Civil War by George Winston Smith

Pharmaceutical Education in the Queen City: 150 years of Service, 1850-2000 by Michael A. Flannery and Dennis B. Worthen

American Women Pharmacists: Contributions to the Profession by Metta Lou Henderson

A History of Nonprescription Product Regulation by W. Steven Pray

Federal Drug Control: The Evolution of Policy and Practice edited by Jonathon Erlen and Joseph F. Spillane

A Social History of Medicines in the Twentieth Century: To Be Taken Three Times a Day by John K. Crellin

Pharmacy in World War II by Dennis B. Worthen

Civil War Pharmacy: A History of Drugs, Drug Supply and Provision, and Therapeutics for the Union and Confederacy by Michael A. Flannery

Dictionary of Pharmacy edited by Dennis B. Worthen

Pharmacy in World War II

Dennis B. Worthen, PhD

Pharmaceutical Products Press®
An Imprint of The Haworth Press, Inc.
New York • London • Oxford

Published by

Pharmaceutical Heritage Editions, a series from Pharmaceutical Products Press®, an imprint of The Haworth Press, Inc., 10 Alice Street, Binghamton, NY 13904-1580.

Cover design by Lora Wiggins.

Cover image, "Serving at Home or in the Armed Forces," from Griffenhagen, G. *150 Years of Caring: A Pictorial History of the American Pharmaceutical Association.* American Pharmacists Association, Washington, DC. 2002. Reprinted with permission.

Library of Congress Cataloging-in-Publication Data

Worthen, Dennis B.
    Pharmacy in World War II / Dennis B. Worthen.
        p. ; cm.—(Pharmaceutical heritage editions)
    Includes bibliographical references and index.
        ISBN 0-7890-1625-7 (case : alk. paper)—ISBN 0-7890-1626-5 (soft : alk. paper)
    1. Pharmacy—United States—History—20th century—Anecdotes. 2. Medicine—United States—History—20th century—Anecdotes. 3. World War II—History—Anecdotes.
    [DNLM: 1. Pharmacy—history—United States—Personal Narratives. 2. History of Medicine, 20th Cent.—United States—Personal Narratives. 3. Military Medicine—history—United States—Personal Narratives. 4. Pharmacists—history—United States—Personal Narratives. 5. War—history—United States—Personal Narratives. UH 423 W932p 2004] I. Title: Pharmacy in World War 2. II. Title: Pharmacy in World War two. III. Title. IV. Pharmaceutical heritage.
    RS61 .W75 2004
    615'.1'097309045—dc22
                                                                        2003016162

To Patti
with thanks and love for making this trip with me

For the pharmacists and pharmacy students
who paid the price

ABOUT THE AUTHOR

Dennis B. Worthen, PhD, is Lloyd Scholar at the Lloyd Library and Museum in Cincinnati, Ohio. He is an adjunct professor at the University of Cincinnati College of Pharmacy, where he teaches the history of pharmacy. He retired from Procter & Gamble Health Care in 1999 after twenty-three years of service, and most recently as Director of Pharmacy Affairs.

Dr. Worthen received a BA from the University of Michigan, and from Case Western Reserve University he earned two MS degrees and a PhD. From 1986 to 1989, he was awarded an Allied Irish Bank visiting professorship at the College of Pharmacy at Queen's University in Belfast, Northern Ireland. In 1996 he received the American Institute of the History of Pharmacy Fischelis Grant for his research on pharmacy in World War II.

Dr. Worthen is the co-author of *Pharmaceutical Education in the Queen City: 150 Years of Service 1850-2000* (Haworth Press), a history of the University of Cincinnati College of Pharmacy. He is the editor of *A Road Map to a Profession's Future: The Millis Study Commission on Pharmacy,* to which he also contributed, and is editor-in-chief of the *Dictionary of Pharmacy.* He has published more than sixty papers in professional journals.

Dr. Worthen is a contributing author for the *International Journal of Pharmaceutical Compounding* and is the author of the "Heroes of Pharmacy" series for the *Journal of the American Pharmaceutical Association.* In 1998, he was the founding co-editor of the Pharmaceutical Heritage book series of Haworth Press, devoted to publishing books covering historical aspects of pharmacy, and is editor-in-chief of Haworth's Pharmaceutical Products Press.

CONTENTS

Foreword

There are but a handful of books that deal with the history of pharmacy in the United States and but a few small institutional histories that have been devoted, as is this book, entirely to developments in the twentieth century. The present text, although its focal point is the impact of World War II on pharmacy, provides us with a comprehensive picture of the organizational, economic, educational, professional, and societal factors—and problems—that molded, and were, American pharmacy in the mid-twentieth century. It is concerned with both civilian and military pharmacy from before Pearl Harbor to the postwar years.

Thus we are provided with an account of the activities of the national professional, trade, and educational institutions of pharmacy, and we follow their goals and development as well as their interactions, agreements, and differences. The roles of the leaders in the pharmacy establishment all are depicted, and their activities, as they are recounted in this book, center on their efforts to gain professional recognition for pharmacy in the military services. These led, eventually, after continuous confrontation with the military—detailed in this text for the first time—to the rather hollow victory of the establishment of the Pharmacy Corps.

The military's contention that all necessary pharmaceutical services could be imparted in ninety days of training or less rankled the pharmacy establishment. The attitude of the military reflected not only the age-long condescension of medical men toward the pharmacist but also the belief that the drugstore was a place of business and the pharmacist a businessman rather than a professional.

The continuous refusal to give any recognition to the trained pharmacist carried over into the Selective Service. This book devotes, for the first time, considerable attention to the impact of the Selective Service beyond its effect on the individual pharmacist and pharmacy student. Selective Service caused the attrition of the number of community pharmacies and had disastrous effects on enrollments in schools of pharmacy. Also brought to attention is the work of the state committees of pharmacists set up to advise Selective Service. These advisory committees played a decisive role in the process of helping to determine the criteria of deferments of pharmacists and the application of these criteria to individual cases. Dr. Worthen has provided, in Appendix II, a list of the members of these advisory committees—pharmacists whose wartime activity and service has previously gone unrecorded.

The war thus had a direct impact on pharmacy and the activities of pharmacists. Scarcities of drugs concerned both the war effort and civilian requirements. Manpower shortages forced many community pharmacies to close down. The meager enrollments in schools of pharmacy caused concern for the future supply of qualified pharmacists. Yet both military and civilian needs were met in the face of these critical times. Moreover, the drugstore played its part in the war effort as a depot for the purchase of war stamps and as a collection site of used tin tubes (and for finding alternatives for the tin tube in dispensing). Perhaps the most visible activity, and certainly the most important, was the response to the call for the pharmacists to clear their shelves of quinine products and to turn them over to the American Pharmaceutical Association for use by the military.

This book had its origin in the responses to Dr. Worthen's call to pharmacists and pharmacy students to tell him of their wartime experiences—civilian and military. In the process Dr. Worthen built a database of almost 11,000 names of pharmacists, pharmacy students, and veterans in pharmacy school. The book is enriched with many personal recollections; each recollection has poignancy about it and a feeling of pride in the support of the war effort. For almost all in the military there is an undercurrent feeling of being underused and unappreciated as professionals as they were assigned to nonpharmaceutical tasks. All, however, give ample evidence of patriotism and self-sacrifice.

It is thus most fitting that the last of the information-laden appendixes is a list of the 131 pharmacists and pharmacy students in the military who died in the war. The list must, of course, bring back sad memories, and I think back to three of my students, barely out of their teens, killed in action in the Battle of the Bulge. I have dedicated my book, *The New Jersey Pharmaceutical Association 1870-1970,* to the memory of Alex Chase, Manfred Keitsch, and Salvatore F. Procopio, in sorrow for their lost humanity and potential. Dr. Worthen has done honor to these three and to the many who did not return to home and pharmacy after the war.

David L. Cowen
Professor Emeritus of History
Rutgers University

Preface

In 1995 a number of commemorations marked the fiftieth anniversary of the end of World War II. Several years earlier I had stumbled across some documentation of the Army Navy "E" Award for production by a pharmaceutical company. One thing led to another, and almost before I knew it Mickey Smith and I had published a short piece on the contributions of the pharmaceutical industry to the war effort. This paper concluded with a call to pharmacists for their memories of the war.[1] I never contemplated that this request would prove to be a life-defining moment.

The first letters I received were from Harvey Mamet, a retired pharmacist in Syracuse, New York:

> My attachment to Pharmacy started at age 13 when I received my Apprentice Certificate from New York State. I graduated from the Buffalo College of Pharmacy in January 1943. It was a wartime graduation with a number of my classmates having gone into the service right after their last exam. After the graduation ceremony I returned to Syracuse and after a few weeks in retail pharmacy, went to work for the Cheplin Biological division of Bristol Labs. There I was the pharmacist involved in pilot plant production of penicillin. In the fall of 1943 I was inducted into the Army and after basic training at Fort Benning, GA, I was sent to Camp Livingston, LA. Even though I was a pharmacy graduate and licensed to practice pharmacy—I was classified as an infantryman. While at Camp Livingston, I continued to be in the infantry even though I requested transfer to the medics. My infantry training kept accelerating with maneuvers, jungle fighting, qualifying on the 60 MM mortar, etc. No matter how hard I tried to get into some medical field, I was told that infantrymen were more valuable than medics!

As it turned out I was shipped overseas to Europe as a mortar man and rifleman in late summer 1944. During the Battle of the Bulge I was one of the many riflemen who were stationed in the woods outside of Paris as a precaution against saboteurs and enemy patrols.

At that point someone must have read my record and saw that I was a pharmacist. My rifle was taken away and I was assigned to the medical detachment of the 143 Infantry regiment in the 36th Division. My new job was as a litter bearer which I don't remember having studied in pharmacy school. Litter bearers had the task of going by jeep as close to the front as possible, then by foot in teams of two men and retrieving the wounded.

One day the battalion surgeon called me in for a demonstration on how to use a morphine Syrette and how to apply Carlisle bandages. After the 20 minute course I was assigned as the medic for I Company, 143rd Infantry. My only "weapon" was the red cross on my helmet. I was fortunate to have had probably more training in how to survive under fire than most of the replacements that came along.

For a time after the 36th division I was with the 47th Armored Battalion of the 1st Armored Division. This was occupation duty and I really had no special assignment so I set up a "pharmacy" in the kitchen of the house that we used for headquarters. There I was able to requisition from medical supply and take from deserted apothecary shops those items I felt necessary. About the only thing I manufactured was Elixir of Terpin Hydrate with Codeine. I soon left out the codeine because the nickname was "GI Gin" and the men didn't need overdoses of codeine.

After VE Day, my division was sent back to the States and I was assigned to the 130th Station Hospital at Heidelberg, Germany. The 130th had a pharmacy; the "pharmacist" was a former truck driver who had a three-month course somewhere on how to run a hospital pharmacy.

Most of my experiences I found were locked away in my memory. Only the 50th anniversary of the war's events has brought them to mind. To be under enemy fire, riding tanks into battle, living in holes and basements, seeing friends killed and wounded, are all terrible memories. Looking at my Combat Medic badge and reading the field order that gave me the award makes the tears flow.[2]

Mamet's letters provided a synopsis of pharmacy from 1941 through 1945. He told of his wartime graduation, civilian work experiences, and then military induction and the frustration of dealing with a military that did not value his education. His letters were engaging and made me want to learn more about pharmacy and pharmacists during the war. This work began thanks to Harvey Mamet.

I could find no comprehensive, contemporary history of pharmacy during the war years. The records of pharmacists in the military and at home were scattered. Many of the state and national pharmacy journals had documented the routines of practice at the home front but these themes had not been gathered and published. Many of the same journals provided glimpses of the men who had left their practices and education to serve in the military, but these insights were likewise scattered. The war years are generally acknowledged as a historic watershed in American history. They certainly were an important time in American pharmacy, but what happened in pharmacy? Where were the records; what were the stories?

In 1996 I applied to the American Institute of the History of Pharmacy for a Fischelis Grant to answer the questions about pharmacy in World War II. The objective was to collect, organize, and disseminate the memories of pharmacists during the World War II period (1941-1945). The application was approved and the project was launched. The national and state pharmacy associations, boards of pharmacy, colleges and schools of pharmacy, and pharmacy publications were contacted and asked for information from their files and help in contacting pharmacists who had served in the military during the war and those who had worked on the home front. Many of those contacted printed notices about the project, now called the Memories Project, and asked pharmacists to contact me.

Over 300 individuals contacted me, and in some cases children or other relatives responded for their deceased loved ones. Some of the respondents shared little beyond the fact that they had served in a particular branch of the Armed Forces and where they went to pharmacy school. Other respondents provided extensive memories of what they

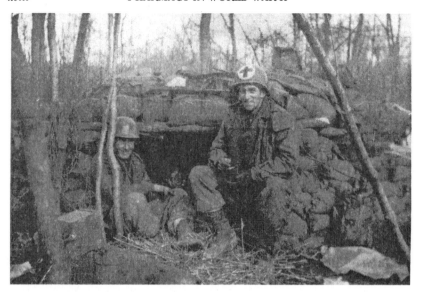

The individual on the left is Harvey Mamet, a 1943 graduate of the Buffalo College of Pharmacy. Mamet, a rifleman during the Battle of the Bulge, later transferred to the Medics where he earned the Combat Medic Badge during the push into Germany. This photo was taken in the Rhine Valley near Drusenheim in February 1945. (*Source:* Memories Project Files.)

did in the military, and some shared memories of the home front. These men and women are listed with gratitude in Appendix IV.

As the letters started arriving, it became clear that collecting letters and printing them was not enough to tell the story of pharmacy. No single letter, or even group of letters, could tell the story of the fight for a pharmacy corps in the Army, the shortages and rationing on the home front, or the military experiences of pharmacists. The letters likewise could not fully tell of manpower shortages, the conservation orders for quinine and tin, or the Selective Service. The letters needed to be put into the broader context of what was happening to and in pharmacy.

What follows is the story of a profession during the conflagration of World War II as recorded in publications, stored in archives, and told by its practitioners. It is not a story of military heroes, although there were some, but the recognition that pharmacists were an integral part of American society. While the pharmaceutical industry was considered an integral part of the profession during the war and many pharmacists played an active part in the research, production, and distribution of new medicines to the troops and the civilians on the home front, their stories are yet to be told. The stories of pharmacists working in the wartime agencies, such as the War Production Board, and regulatory agencies are also yet to be fully explored.

Author's Note

I have chosen to use the terms of the historical period of World War II rather than artificially modernize them. While these terms may sound unfamiliar or dated to today's reader, they accurately reflect the memories and the literature of the period. Thus the terms *druggist* and *drugstore* are used when they were used in the original materials. Images of the period overwhelmingly show that the retail establishments were called drugstores, not pharmacies. This usage also manages to avoid the confusion that arises over the current term, *pharmacy,* which can relate to both the physical setting and the profession.

I have also chosen to retain the pronouns relating to the masculine gender when writing about pharmacists of the period—for the profession was mostly made up of males. World War II created the opportunity for women to join the profession in greater numbers than ever before. Frequently, the term used to describe female pharmacists during the war period was *girl pharmacist.*

I have also, where appropriate, used the racial and ethnic terms of the period. This is not to justify or explain some terms that are not popular in today's climate of political correctness. They were, however, in common use and are reflective of the period.

All citations identified as "Memories Project Files" are correspondence and other materials provided to the author by the individual named. The files are in the possession of the author and, upon completion of the project, will be deposited with the American Institute of the History of Pharmacy in Madison, Wisconsin.

Pharmacy organizations are referred to by the acronyms of the period:

AACP	American Association of Colleges of Pharmacy
ACA	American College of Apothecaries
ACPE	American Council on Pharmaceutical Education
AFPE	American Foundation for Pharmaceutical Education

APhA   American Pharmaceutical Association
ASHP   American Society of Hospital Pharmacists
NABP   National Association of Boards of Pharmacy
NARD   National Association of Retail Druggists
NWDA   National Wholesale Druggists Association

Acknowledgments

I am deeply indebted to the men and women who shared their memories.

I am grateful to the many pharmacy journal editors, deans and faculty at virtually every U.S. college of pharmacy, state pharmacy association executives, and the directors of the state boards of pharmacy who graciously responded to my requests for information, memories, and documents.

This work was supported in part through the American Institute of the History of Pharmacy American Institute of the History of Pharmacy Fischelis Grant, "Pharmacists in Wartime: Memories of a Profession" (1996). I am grateful to the institute not only for the grant but also for the encouragement to undertake and complete the work.

The board and staff of the Lloyd Library were extraordinarily supportive in the preparation of this work. In addition to an institutional home, they provided many support services that were essential to the completion of the research and writing.

Special thanks are due to John Graham and John Hendricks and the entire staff in the Public Documents Department at the Public Library of Cincinnati and Hamilton County. Their ability to find obscure materials was uncanny, and all were superb to work with.

Staff in the offices of the surgeons general of the Army and Navy were helpful in locating materials relating to the development of pharmacy in their respective branches.

John Parascandola was ever willing to respond to my questions about the Public Health Service, the Merchant Marine, and the Coast Guard.

My thanks to Greg Higby and Elaine Stroud for facilitating the work in the Kremer Files at the American Institute of the History of Pharmacy.

The reference staff of the Wisconsin Historical Society were most helpful in working through the collections that are housed in their facility, including the Fischelis papers and the archives of the American Association of Colleges of Pharmacy.

George Griffenhagen facilitated using the American Pharmaceutical Association files and willingly shared his encyclopedic knowledge of the association and its leaders.

A number of individuals responded with good cheer and no sign of visible exasperation as question followed question: Rita Benischek (University of Oklahoma), Clarence Ueda (University of Nebraska), Ken Kirk (St. Louis College of Pharmacy), and Metta Lou Henderson (Ohio Northern University).

Special thanks are due to Mickey Smith and Richard Jackson who co-authored papers on World War II topics with me. Mickey and I worked together on several early publications dealing with pharmaceuticals in World War II. Richard Jackson and I worked through some of the economic factors of drugstores during the war years.

Grateful acknowledgment is made to the American Pharmaceutical Association *(Journal of the American Pharmaceutical Association),* the American Institute of the History of Pharmacy *(Pharmacy in History),* and the Albany College of Pharmacy *(PostScript)* for permission to draw on materials published in their journals.

The following organizations were gracious in their permission to reproduce images from their publications: New Jersey Pharmacists Association, the *New Jersey Journal of Pharmacy;* American Pharmaceutical Association, *Journal of the American Pharmaceutical Association;* National Community Pharmacists Association, *NARD Journal;* North Carolina Association of Pharmacists, *Carolina Journal of Pharmacy;* and Albany College of Pharmacy, *PostScript.* The Marvin Sampson Center of the University of the Sciences in Philadelphia also provided permission for the Quinine V certificate photograph. The University of Florida College of Pharmacy and Wanda Cowart Ebersole granted permission for the use of photo and caption of the dispensing laboratory.

I am deeply indebted to the individuals who read the manuscript and provided their expertise and guidance: David L. Cowen, professor emeritus at Rutgers University; Michael Flannery, associate director for Historical Collections of the Lister Hill Library; and Glenn Sonnedecker, professor emeritus of the University of Wisconsin.

My partner in this work, as in all of my work, has been Patti Lynn Worthen. She has been an active and willing research partner as she scanned journals, photocopied, and provided her own special editing skills to every page.

As should be the case, the responsibility for any errors is mine.

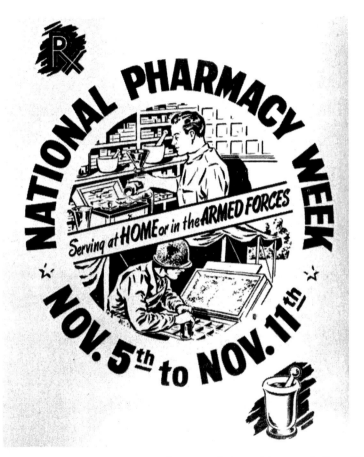

This image of a pharmacist compounding prescriptions at home or in the military was the center of the Pharmacy Week poster in the fall of 1944. The image was widely produced in professional journals. Posters and other materials were distributed to retail pharmacies to promote Pharmacy Week to the public. (*Source:* From Griffenhagen, G. [2002]. *150 Years of Caring: A Pictorial History of the American Pharmaceutical Association.* Washington DC: American Pharmacists Association. Reprinted with permission.)

Chapter 1

Prologue:
Prewar Pharmacy Practice, 1940-1941

> Pharmacy will meet the demands whatever they may be, as she
> has in the past—come war, pestilence or flood. . . . The com-
> bined resources of our profession are at our Government's dis-
> posal. Pharmacy has never failed.[1]

The summaries of the 1941 annual meetings of the national pharmacy associations provide a picture of a profession poised between
the concerns of war and peace. The reports of routine, peace-time issues such as education, standards, and federal regulations were punc-
tuated with concerns about shortages of medicines and manpower
and the status of pharmacists in the military. It was recognized that
pharmacy would be called upon to do its share when the United States
entered the conflict that had already engulfed much of the world.

RETAIL PHARMACY

The druggist and the drugstore were an integral part of the American
neighborhood in the years leading up to the war. In 1938 Thornton
Wilder commented in *Our Town* that everyone in Grover's Corners,
New Hampshire, went into Mr. Morgan's drugstore every day and set
the scene for George Gibbs and Emily Webb to discover their love over
ice cream sodas.[2] Robert Nixon, in *Corner Druggist,* published in
1941, provided a vignette of the man behind the prescription counter:

> Father's position was at once the most obscure and most impor-
> tant in the community; he was engaged in work which, from the
> beginning of recorded time, has snared the imagination and yet
> of which few people have any knowledge; he performed the

greatest service for the lowest pay—he was a neighborhood druggist . . . Every man plodding through a sixteen-hour day, handling the elixirs and tinctures which had the properties of life and death in them, . . . the doctor's right hand, the father confessor of the neighborhood, the guardian of the public health.[3]

Most pharmacists were engaged in retail practice, largely in independent pharmacies. In 1939 approximately 79 percent of the stores were independents, 7 percent chains, and the remainder members of co-ops.[4] The prescription area in the average drugstore was staffed by one or two pharmacists. *Lilly Digest* data for 1941 show that the number of prescriptions per day for the reporting stores ranged from as few as one to more than forty and that the average prescription prices ranged from $1.04 for small-volume stores to $0.93 for large-volume units. Only 9 percent of the reporting stores showed an operating loss, down from 14 percent the prior year, while 56 percent reported a profit of 5 percent or more on sales; over 60 percent of the stores had annual sales volume of less than $20,000.[5]

APhA's President Evans, in his 1941 inaugural address, identified that one of the organization's greatest challenges was to reach out to the retail pharmacists of the nation. He noted that there were 130,000 pharmacists working in 60,000 drugstores, most of which were one-man operations.[6] Eighty percent of the licensed pharmacists in the United States were employed as retail pharmacists, and they commonly occupied a position of leadership and trust in both rural and urban areas. The pharmacist was an educated professional, one who was sought for counsel in many communities. Their stores provided a convenient gathering place for communities and neighborhoods and provided an environment where public sentiment was crystallized.[7]

EDUCATION

Concern about maintaining the standards of pharmacy education was high. The mandatory four-year bachelor's degree program had only begun in 1932. There was a concern that a continued manpower shortage would result in moving away from the standard. The lingering effects of the Great Depression, the implementation of the four-year degree, and the military draft were noted as factors in the manpower concern.

In 1940-1941, fifty-eight colleges of pharmacy held membership in the American Association of Colleges of Pharmacy. At this time colleges did not have to hold membership to become accredited. Total enrollment in the member colleges was 8,410, with an entering class of 2,904. Of the entering students almost 30 percent had previous college experience. In 1941 the member colleges graduated 1,465 with a bachelor of science degree and sixty-seven with graduate degrees.[8]

The American Council on Pharmaceutical Education was established in 1932 as the organization responsible for the accreditation of pharmacy schools. The original sponsoring organizations were the National Association of Boards of Pharmacy, the American Association of Colleges of Pharmacy, and the American Pharmaceutical Association. Standards for accreditation included the following factors: college administration and organization, curriculum, faculty credentials, instructional equipment with emphasis on laboratory and library facilities, and finances.[9] As of 1939, sixty-one of the sixty-eight operating colleges had started the application process for accreditation.[10]

On September 16, 1940, the Burke-Wadsworth Bill passed Congress and became law as the Selective Training and Service Act. One month later the registration period for all males between the ages of twenty-one to thirty-five began, and thirteen days later, on October 29, 1940, Secretary of War Stimson drew the capsule containing the first number of the draft.[11] The Selective Training and Service Act established the length of military service at one year, at the end of which there was an obligation of ten years in the Army reserves.[12] Any exemption from service was based on the decision of the individual's draft board. Pharmacists and pharmacy students did not have a blanket exemption. Students could be exempted to complete their current year of academic work, and individual pharmacists could be exempted if their service to the community was considered to be necessary to the public health. The fact that a pharmacist was in a one-man store was not sufficient to qualify for an exemption, however, unless the loss of the pharmaceutical services would be significant to the community.[13]

Support for student finances and scholarships was a constant concern. College administrators looked to other pharmacy groups—including manufacturers and wholesalers—to help resolve this issue. The National Drug Trade Conference, a loose association of nine industry and professional associations, was aware of the manpower and financial concerns of the colleges and the need to develop an ongoing funding source.* In late 1941 the conference agreed to set up a foundation that would raise funds for the purpose of supporting pharmaceutical education.[14] The American Foundation for Pharmaceutical Education was incorporated in 1942.

An awareness was growing of the need for refresher courses—the forerunner of continuing professional education. The need to keep pharmacists current with the changing world of practice was noted in both APhA President Charles Evans' and President-Elect Bernard V. Christensen's addresses. A number of state associations had offered conferences and short courses in the past, but these did not reach the large numbers of pharmacists that needed them. Many colleges started offering programs in the late 1930s; the program at Purdue was probably the most notable.[15] Wisconsin took the lead in utilizing the George-Dreen Act for vocational training by establishing an extension program that provided ongoing education to pharmacists throughout the state. A tentative program was drawn up by an advisory committee from AACP, APhA, NABP, and NARD to expand the Wisconsin experience to other states. Programs were divided into three areas: (1) selling pharmaceutical service, (2) store management, operations, and sales direction, and (3) merchandising by departments. Pharmacists who completed a year's course would be awarded a certificate, and five certificates would qualify the participant for a national diploma that would be signed by the secretaries of AACP, APhA, NABP, and NARD.[16]

MANPOWER

Manpower shortages became a pervasive and unifying concern of pharmacy. There were scant data to prove a shortage of licensed pharmacists, and this lack affected decisions and activities between the

---

*The associations were the American Drug Manufacturers Association, American Pharmaceutical Association, American Pharmaceutical Manufacturers Association, Federal Wholesale Druggists Association, National Association of Boards of Pharmacy, National Association of Retail Druggists, National Wholesale Druggists' Association, Proprietary Association, and American Association of Colleges of Pharmacy.

profession and governmental agencies—especially Selective Service.[17] Manpower concerns grew on the local and state levels as retail pharmacies closed or converted to general merchandise retailers because of insufficient numbers of registered pharmacists. Manpower issues also affected the colleges and schools of pharmacy; enrollments fell as the young men entered the military.[18]

Inconsistent numbers were given for pharmacists practicing in the retail setting and for the total number licensed in the United States. In his 1940 presidential installation address, Evans stated that there were 130,000 retail pharmacists. The *Journal of the American Pharmaceutical Association,* Practical Pharmacy Edition, was intended to serve the 115,000 pharmacists in retail practice.[19] The best estimate of the number of pharmacists, however, probably came from the 1940 Census of Occupational Employment, since each pharmacist was counted only once, while state board compilations counted an individual in each state where he or she held a license. State numbers also included those licensed pharmacists who were working in other occupations, or retired, and sometimes even dead. The 1940 census reported 81,924 practitioners licensed in the forty-eight states and the District of Columbia, including 78,708 men and 3,216 women; the total number of drugstores operating in 1939 was 57,903. Many state boards did not maintain gender records for licensed pharmacists, and estimates of women in pharmacy ranged from 3.1 to 5.6 percent of the total licensed practitioners.[20] The census also provided a count of 8,945 pharmacy students in 1940 (7,945 men and 1,000 women) and a graduating class of 1,511.[21] This number fell far short of the estimated 2,100 pharmacists needed to replace those who died or retired each year.

PHARMACY CORPS

As part of his presidential address, Charles Evans urged pharmacy to demand that Congress create a separate, commissioned Pharmacy Corps. The issue of pharmacists' status in the military had long been a struggle between organized pharmacy and the Army. Since the Army would not make the necessary accommodations, an alternative legislative strategy was devised. During his incoming APhA presidential address in 1941, Bernard V. Christensen continued his predecessors' emphasis on the status of pharmacists in the military, stating that

> the man in uniform is entitled to a choice of drugs and medicines adapted to his individual needs, he is entitled to pure and efficient drugs, he is entitled to skillful and accurate compounding just as is the man in civilian clothes.[22]

The association passed two resolutions involving pharmacists in the military. The first, Resolution 10, instructed the Committee on the Status of Pharmacists in the Government Service to seek congressional action that would assure proper supervision of pharmaceutical services for the protection of the Armed Forces. The second, Resolution 22, noted that the compounding of prescriptions in civilian life was restricted to trained, licensed professionals and requested that only licensed pharmacists be assigned to compound in the military. The resolution focused solely on the issue of licensure and safety; copies were sent to the surgeon general of the Army and to the Military Affairs Committees in both houses of Congress.[23]

PRACTICE STANDARDS

NABP took action in 1940 on several important practice standards. The first action, effective in 1944, was to establish graduation from an ACPE institution as a prerequisite for licensure reciprocity between the states. The second action was to establish new standards for the practical experience requirements (effective 1943), notably defining a year as fifty-two weeks of at least forty-eight hours per week under the direct supervision of a registered pharmacist. Six months of the experience had to be in a hospital or retail pharmacy that filled a minimum of 1,000 prescriptions per year.[24]

A joint committee of NABP, AACP, and APhA continued the effort to modernize the state pharmacy practice laws, which many considered antiquated and unresponsive to either practice or public health needs. The Committee on Modernization of Pharmacy Laws prepared a Model Practice Act that could be used by state legislatures. The Model Practice Act was based on the fundamental principal that medicines were essential to public health and that adequate safeguards should be provided for the safe handling and use of potent products. One element of the model was that all steps in the preparation and distribution of medicines should be controlled. This included controlling the manufacturer and wholesaler as well as the pharmacist. The Model Practice Act also considered physicians, dentists, and veterinarians as performing a pharmacist's duties when dispensing directly to patients and should, therefore, be subject to the same regulations and controls as the pharmacist. The committee believed that pharmacists supported the tone and purpose of the act; however, there was little support by state legislators, who often failed to recognize the intrinsic merits of the profession.[25]

SHORTAGES

Shortages of USP standard ingredients were being addressed by the pharmacopoeia in 1941. Supplies of some items, such as cod-liver oil and oil of lavender, were being restricted by war conditions in Europe and Asia. In a number of cases alternatives were being developed, such as the use of domestically grown belladonna leaf to replace imported belladonna. Some products, such as oil of rose, could be eliminated from USP formulations without creating a medical problem. The commissioner of narcotics requested state agencies to curtail the availability of all exempt narcotics, except for low doses of codeine, in order to conserve the supply of narcotics already in the country.[26] Prior to the end of 1941 the government identified a number of essential drugs and authorized stockpile levels, such as 50,000 pounds of aconite root, 200,000 pounds of belladonna leaves and 60,000 pounds of roots, 200,000 pounds of ergot of rye, and 675,000 pounds of red squill. With the exception of ergot of rye with 31 percent and quinine with 84 percent of the objective amounts in hand, there were no appreciable stockpiles.[27]

DECEMBER 7, 1941

Pharmacy's world on the eve of December 7, 1941, was concerned with a number of pressing needs and concerns. Manpower shortages, perceived or real, were a concern as enrollment in the colleges remained low and a number of the younger men were called into the military with the peacetime draft. The conflict in Asia and Europe made itself felt in the shortages of some prescription ingredients and tin. All of these global issues became much more real and personal on December 7 as recalled by Edmund E. Ehlke. Ehlke, a 1939 graduate of the University of Washington, was a pharmacist at the Queen's Hospital in Honolulu in December 1941. He was awakened on the morning of December 7 with the news of the Japanese attack:

By the time that I arrived at Queen's the floor was covered with dead or dying people waiting for medical care. Queen's had a total of six interns plus our medical staff and everyone was extremely busy attempting to save lives. Our patient load was from the citizenry of Honolulu who had been injured by strafing or bombs. Fortunately for Hawaii, the Queen's hospital was one of the few hospitals in Honolulu with a fairly good supply of morphine sulfate. One of my first assignments was to make up 30 ML bottles of morphine sulfate in the strength of one-half grain per ML. Nearly all of our supply went to Hickam and Pearl Harbor as that was the scene of the greatest need for analgesics due to the tremendous devastation and need. At one point in the morning, the electricity was cut and myself and both Filipinos and Japanese orderlies carried patients on stretchers up a winding stairway to the fourth floor where we had an emergency generator set up for the doctors doing surgery. Our Baxter Solution, which we used for intravenous administration, was stored in the basement below the pharmacy and I was busy most of the day carrying cases from the basement to the surgical department. I also prepared several gallons of a burn solution consisting of a mixture of sodium sulfanilamide, tannic acid, and resorcinol, which we sprayed on the body of the badly burned victims, using the old Hudson bug sprayer. As pharmacist, I was on duty at Queen's on a 24-hour basis, sleeping catch as catch can in the old intern shack. It was about two weeks before I was able to return home.

As there was no blood bank at this time, all of the liquor that was confiscated by the Honolulu Police Department in raids of poker games during the blackout following the "blitz," was brought to the pharmacy at Queen's as we had a locked cement vault for our storage of ethyl alcohol and narcotics. Whenever an individual was fined by the Provost Marshall for some misdemeanor, the fine imposed was five dollars or a pint of blood. Those giving a pint of blood were given two ounces of whatever liquor was available in our vault, thus Dr. Forrest J. Pinkerton started our blood bank.[28]

Chapter 2

Pharmacy Education

The old methods to which we are accustomed are not just fading; they are shattered. Traditional modes of life are not being gradually transformed; they are suddenly upset. Old ways of thinking—well, they are just blasted out.[1]

Thus H. Evert Kendig, immediate past president of the American Association of the Colleges of Pharmacy, responded to questions from Rudolph Kuever, the incoming president, and Charles H. Rogers, the chairman of the Executive Committee, concerning the need to accelerate the four-year pharmacy curriculum in 1942. Kendig was acknowledging that the changes the war would bring to the colleges* were likely to be revolutionary rather than evolutionary.

THE COLLEGES

By 1942 there were sixty-eight colleges of pharmacy operating; sixty-five had applied for accreditation or were already accredited by the American Council on Pharmaceutical Education. Fifty-nine colleges held membership in the American Association of Colleges of Pharmacy (see Appendix I).[2] Several universities discontinued their colleges of pharmacy just before the beginning of the war; the University of Notre Dame was closed in 1939 and Valparaiso in Indiana and North Pacific College in Oregon both closed in 1941. At the beginning of the war years, a college did not have to be accredited by ACPE or a member of AACP in order to provide instruction in phar-

---

*In the spirit of simplicity, I use the term *college* to represent all educational institutions unless a specific institution is being referred to, in which case the proper term is used.

macy; graduates were still eligible to take the state board exam for licensure since the ultimate authority for the requirements for state licensure rested with the individual states.

THE CURRICULUM

Pharmacy education had moved to a mandatory four-year bachelor of science curriculum with the entering freshman class of 1932. A standardized curriculum was developed by the National Pharmaceutical Syllabus Committee made up of representatives of the American Pharmaceutical Association, the American Association of Colleges of Pharmacy, and the National Association of Boards of Pharmacy. This curriculum set standards for which materials should be taught in the colleges in order for the graduates to pass the state boards' examinations and enter practice. Thus the curriculum established a set of expectations for the profession at large (see Table 2.1).

The fourth edition of the *Pharmaceutical Syllabus* was published in 1932. While there was latitude in which courses could be offered by individual colleges and how the subject was to be taught, there was still the recognition of the need for a national standard for those licensed to practice pharmacy. The purposes of the *Syllabus* as explained in the preface included:

> (1) to present the essentials that should be included in the college curricula; (2) to outline subjects of a professional or applied character in such a way as to foster a degree of uniformity which will tend to equalize the training of pharmacists sufficiently to assure their professional capability irrespective of the geographic location of the teaching institution or its educational policy; and (3) to give in the several outlines such attention to detail as will guide boards in framing their examinations.[3]

The fourth edition of the *Pharmaceutical Syllabus* was organized into two sections; the first was made up of professional and applied subjects and the second consisted of the basic subjects, predominantly chemistry. The student was required to complete a minimum of 3,000 clock hours of instruction over four years; over 2,300 hours were in required subjects.

TABLE 2.1. Four-Year Curriculum*

Section I. Professional and Applied Subjects	Required Subjects			Optional Subjects		
	Didactic Hours	Laboratory Hours	Total Hours	Didactic Hours	Laboratory Hours	Total Hours
Pharmacy subjects	448	320	768	—	96	96
Pharmaceutical chemistry subjects	48	64	112	128	192	320
Pharmacognosy subjects	64	64	128	16	64	80
Pharmacology subjects	96	32	128	—	—	—
Allied science subjects	80	64	144	48	48	96
Business subjects	—	—	—	96	128	224
Total hours	736	544	1,280	288	528	816

Section II. Basic Subjects	Required Subjects			Optional Subjects		
	Didactic Hours	Laboratory Hours	Total Hours	Didactic Hours	Laboratory Hours	Total Hours
Natural sciences	224	320	544	64	128	194
Biological sciences	112	112	224	32	64	96
Economics	96	—	96	—	—	—
Languages	96	—	96	96	—	96
Mathematics	96	—	96	—	—	—
Total hours	624	432	1,056	192	192	386

Source: National Pharmaceutical Syllabus Committee (1932). *The Pharmaceutical Syllabus: Outlining the Course of Instruction for the Degree of Bachelor of Science in Pharmacy (B.S. Phar.),* Fourth Edition, p. 17.

*Not less than 3,000 hours are to be selected from this table.

THE FACULTY

The constitution of the American Association of Colleges of Pharmacy included a section on the composition and background of the teaching staff of a member college. The criteria included such considerations as at least one full-time individual at the professorial level as well as the education and training of the faculty. Teaching schedules were not to exceed sixteen hours a week and laboratories should not exceed thirty students, although there could be more in lectures.[4]

A 1944 editorial by Hugh Muldoon in the *American Journal of Pharmaceutical Education* questioned the availability of faculty to teach in the accelerated courses. Muldoon stated that teaching staffs had been decreased by individuals leaving the colleges for military service or work in other fields. He also noted that many colleges were releasing teachers because there were fewer students to teach. At issue, however, was the question of retaining good teachers for the postwar period and the necessity of preparing the best students to pursue a teaching career.[5]

In the 1944 annual report of the American Council of Pharmaceutical Education, only a small loss of faculty was noted. The largest number of faculty losses came from the ranks of the teaching assistants, with the explanatory comment that with the decreased enrollments their services were not essential.[6] However, the best perspective of the impact on faculty levels during the war is provided by a survey undertaken for the American Foundation for Pharmaceutical Education at the beginning of 1945. The survey showed that the faculty ranks of sixty accredited colleges had decreased from a prewar level of 788 to 644 (down 18 percent). Not all of the faculty losses were due to leave; some were the result of death, retirement, or resignation. Only sixty-six faculty were noted as being on leave for the duration of the war (see Table 2.2).[7] At least two deans were on leave and serving with the military. William Paul Briggs, the dean of the George Washington University School of Pharmacy, was in the Bureau of Medicine and Surgery of the Navy. Briggs was a 1928 graduate of the pharmacy school at George Washington University. After graduation he owned his own drugstore before rejoining the school as a faculty member and becoming dean in 1932.* Lieutenant Colonel James H. Kidder, a physician, was the dean of the Fordham College of Pharmacy; he served with the Army in the European Theater of Operations.[8] Some who did not join the military were assigned to research duties as civilians working for the military or with bodies such as the National Research Council.

---

*After the war, W. Paul Briggs became the director of pharmacy for the Veterans Administration. In 1951 he became the head of the American Foundation for Pharmaceutical Education.

TABLE 2.2. Faculty Wartime Losses

Discipline	Prewar	1945	Loss	Leave for the Duration
Pharmaceutical botany/ pharmacognosy	149	117	32	12
Pharmaceutical chemistry	271	225	46	24
Pharmacology	123	112	11	9
Pharmacy	245	190	55	21
Totals	788	644	144 (18%)	66

Rank	Prewar	1945	Loss	Leave for the Duration
Professor	229	209	20	11
Associate professor	83	79	4	7
Assistant professor	117	115	2	21
Instructors	161	116	45	14
Assistants	141	94	47	13
Teaching fellows	39	10	29	2
Research fellows	18	21	+3	0
Totals	788	644	144	68

Source: DuMez, A. G. (1945). "Report on Need for Graduate Work in Pharmaceutical Subjects Prepared for the American Foundation for Pharmaceutical Education." *American Journal of Pharmaceutical Education,* 9:363-370.

Additional pressures were on the faculty members who remained in the schools during the war. They were teaching in a year-round program and taking up the slack for the faculty who had left for the military or other occupations. In some cases the salaries for those teaching in the accelerated programs were increased. Ohio State, for example, increased its budget 12 percent to accommodate the addition of a summer quarter.[9] In a number of schools the faculty were also called upon to take part in research programs that were important to the war effort. The National Research Council was concerned with the potential shortage of ergot which was used for the treatment of shock and some forms of asthma, as well as its familiar use in labor to produce uterine contractions.

At the University of Michigan a research team headed by Professor Frederick Blicke obtained funding from Eli Lilly; Parke, Davis and Company; and the university to develop possible synthetic substitutes. A second team at Michigan was approached by the Medical Division of the National Research Council to develop a vehicle for the use of sulfas in burns that would reduce the toxicity associated with the tannic acid vehicle.[10] Even before Pearl Harbor there was a shortage of belladonna and other botanical products. R. L. McMurray at Washington State University led a project to determine the feasibility of growing belladonna commercially in the Pacific Northwest.[11]

Pharmacognosy faculty at the University of Minnesota were engaged in a phytochemical and pharmacological study of Indian medicinal plants sponsored by the Department of Agriculture.[12] Pharmacy faculty at Purdue increased the efforts of the manufacturing laboratory and with the efforts of the students prepared many of the pharmaceuticals used by the health services in the university.[13]

Twenty-six schools were offering some form of continuing education, or extension, courses before the war. This number dropped precipitously and by 1942 only a few scattered programs remained. The decline in numbers was due in part to the increased teaching loads imposed by the needs of the accelerated programs. However, other factors included the inability of pharmacists to get away from their stores and problems with travel.[14]

THE STUDENTS

In the academic 1941-1942 year there were 2,546 new students entering the member colleges of AACP. This represented a decline of over 12 percent from the previous year. The explanation for this decrease was seen largely as a consequence of the draft and the appeal of high salaries in war industries. The total enrollment for member colleges was 7,961, also a decrease from the previous year. There were 1,527 graduates with a bachelor's degree at the end of the academic year, thirty-eight with a master's degree, and seventeen with a doctorate. The demographics of the 1941-1942 entering class provide a profile of the average school and student. Of the entering students 723 had previous college work and fifty-five already had degrees. Most of those had bachelor-level degrees (forty-six of the total) and several individuals had non-BS pharmacy degrees (pharmacy graduate [PhG] and pharmaceutical chemist [PhC]). Almost 58 percent of the entering students did not have any prior drugstore experience before entering college. Over 16 percent of the entering class, or 419, were women; this was an increase of over 17 percent from the previous year.[15]

Enrollment impact varied regionally. For example, an article in the *Pacific Drug Review* reported a 17.23 percent national decline of pharmacy students enrolled in the fall of 1942 while the schools of the Pacific Slope reported a decline of 21.3 percent. One of the Pa-

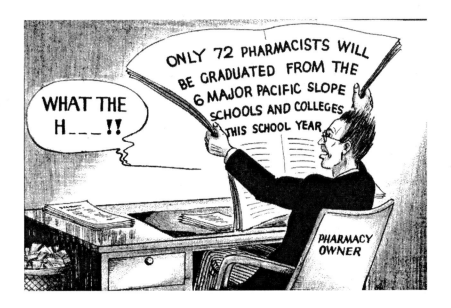

As the war continued, enrollment in pharmacy schools continued to decline. In many cases the student body was made up of men under age eighteen, men classified as 4-F, and women. In January 1944 the outlook was bleak for new pharmacists; most of the men graduating would go into the military immediately after graduation. (*Source: Pacific Drug Review* [1944] 56:23. Photo courtesy of the Lloyd Library and Museum.)

cific Coast schools had only sixteen freshmen enrolled and another reported a drop of total enrollment due to the forced removal of twenty-six Japanese American (Nisei) students by the U.S. government.[16]

The entire issue of student deferment was in a continuous state of shift as is evidenced by the experience of Charles Braucher. Braucher was a student at the Philadelphia College of Pharmacy when the student body was assembled to listen to the radio coverage of President Roosevelt's address to Congress asking for a declaration of war. In 1942 the sophomores and juniors met with an Army captain whose purpose was to increase enrollment in the Army Reserves which would allow the men to graduate before being ordered to active duty. Twenty-eight students, many of them in pharmacy, joined without bothering to read or comprehend the fine print, which stated that the students could still be called up if there was a declaration of national emergency. Within weeks the secretary of war declared a national emergency and all twenty-eight were called into active duty at the end of the semester. Many of the students, including Braucher, were sent to Fort Robertson for basic training and then to the Army Specialized Training Program for a six-month course in engineering. Braucher returned to the Philadelphia College of Pharmacy on the GI Bill at the end of his military service.[17]

By July 1943 the strain of reduced enrollments was being felt in many areas. A survey noted that there were only six graduates with a BS in pharmacy at the University of Toledo, five at the University of Buffalo, and none in Florida. A few schools fared somewhat better with Louisville graduating twenty-one, the University of Maryland twenty-seven, and the Cincinnati College of Pharmacy thirty-two.[18] In the fall of 1943 the total enrollment for AACP colleges was 3,546—2,404 men and 1,142 women. Of the men, 348 were under eighteen years of age and 356 were classified by their draft boards as 4-Fs (see Table 2.3).[19] Selective Service used a classification system that ranged from 1 = A, available immediately for service, to 4-F, not eligible for medical reasons. What was happening was illustrated by the experience of Harry Clark who began his pharmacy school education at the Albany College of Pharmacy in the summer of 1943. He and all of his male classmates received a draft call by the end of the year.[20]

TABLE 2.3. College Enrollment in AACP Colleges

	New Students	Total Enrollment	Women	BS Graduates
1940-1941	2,904	8,410	356	1,465
1941-1942	2,546	7,961	419	1,527
1942-1943	2,047	6,935	1,203	1,583
1943-1944	1,669	3,546	1,142	1,162
1944-1945		3,349	1,599*	587*
1945-1946		5,005†	2,020†	

Source: Data taken from the Annual Reports of the Executive Committee of the American Association of Colleges of Pharmacy and published annually in the *American Journal of Pharmaceutical Education.* This underreports the total numbers of students since schools not holding AACP memberships, even though accredited, were excluded. AACP files, American Institute of the History of Pharmacy Collection housed at the Wisconsin Historical Society, Madison, Wisconsin.* 1944-1945 enrollment data from unpublished data RG 293, Box 38, f8; †enrollment data as of September 1945 RG 293, Box 38, f7.

All of the colleges struggled to continue operating in a period when student enrollments were sharply reduced. Smaller faculties due to many leaving for the military or other war-related services compounded the problem. One Massachusetts college, the Boston School of Pharmacy, suspended its operations from 1943 until 1946. (The school was renamed New England College of Pharmacy in 1949.)

ACCELERATION

One of the first reactions to Pearl Harbor in the academic world was the consideration of accelerated programs that would allow for early graduation of students. On December 16, 1941, the Association of American Medical Colleges recommended that its member colleges consider accelerating the medical course to a year-round system that would result in shortening the course to three years. Within weeks President Kuever of the AACP solicited input from the colleges to determine what course of action pharmacy education should pursue. Kuever laid out three options for the deans to consider. The first was to accelerate the programs so that the average student would have the possibility of finishing course work before being drafted. (At the beginning of 1942, Selective Service was authorized to draft men between the ages of twenty-one and thirty-six.) The second option was to shorten the course to a three-year program. This option was seen as a step back that neither the potential students nor the accrediting bodies of the American Council on Pharmaceutical Education and the state boards of pharmacy would be likely to accept. The third option was to wait and do nothing. As part of the "President's Bulletin Number 5," Kuever raised a number of issues. These ranged from the impact of acceleration on facilities and faculties, to the students' ability to finance their education without summer employment, to the need for state boards to license younger graduates.[21] The responses of twenty deans were included as part of Kuever's "President's Bulletin Number 6." The consensus was that there should be no retreat from the bachelor's degree program. Most of the schools had made no decision concerning acceleration, perhaps because of the perception that there was no current shortage of pharmacists on the home front.[22]

There was some debate over the rationale for moving to a twelve-month academic calendar. The basic questions were whether such a move would result in any additional pharmacists being graduated and whether additional pharmacists were needed or even good for pharmacy. At the March 1942 District 1 meeting, Leslie Barrett of the University of Connecticut College of Pharmacy raised the point that the pool of applicants was probably fixed and that the acceleration of the academic year would not result in a greater number of graduates. The only change would be that students could graduate a year earlier. Barrett also addressed trying to graduate more students at the expense of the quality of the graduates. He concluded his argument that it would be better to "have fewer graduate now than to later find ourselves in the backwash wallowing in the dregs of our own folly."[23]

A number of deans had questioned whether there was any shortage of registered pharmacists for professional duties. Some expressed the sentiment that there were too many drugstores and that pharmacists were frequently spending a great deal of their time on nonprofessional duties. Dean Lester Hayman of the University of West Virginia stated that there was a shortage of pharmacists for current stores but that there were more stores than needed to provide heath services. Dean Forest Goodrich of the University of Washington voiced the opposite point of view, exclaiming that the shortage of pharmacists was already great.[24] On January 30, 1942, A. G. DuMez, dean of the Maryland College of Pharmacy and the secretary of the American Council on Pharmaceutical Education, wrote to Rufus Lyman, the editor of the *American Journal of Pharmaceutical Education,* with great passion on the issue of manpower shortages. DuMez recapitulated the findings of the government that there was not a national shortage of pharmacists. Other surveys found that pharmacists were spending one-half or less of their time on professional activities. DuMez quoted a letter from the Virginia director of Selective Service that pharmacists should be engaged in professional duties rather than nonprofessional activities and that some states might have to change their practice acts to allow prescriptions to be filled in a centralized location manned by registered pharmacists. DuMez added:

I would be concerned with the number of pharmacy graduates being turned out by our colleges of pharmacy, if it were not for the fact that we still have in the field many more pharmacists than are actually needed to give the public adequate pharmaceutical service. However, it is my opinion that we can go on at the present rate for another ten years before we will reach the level where it will be advisable to make real effort to increase the number of students in our schools of pharmacy. I am hoping that the Government will actually do for pharmacy what some of us have been trying to accomplish for the last twenty years, at least. If we can just prevent the commercial interests, as represented by the National Wholesale Druggists' Association, the Proprietary Association of America and the chain stores from getting control and forcing us to produce more pharmacy graduates, I can see a great future for pharmacy. Please, however, do not quote me in this instance as I already have enough fights on my hands.[25]

On February 16, 1942, the Executive Committee of AACP approved an accelerated course for the duration of hostilities provided that accelerated programs maintain the quality and extent of instruction. All but one school approved the committee's action. In March, twenty-five schools announced that they would accelerate their programs effective the summer of 1942; twenty-nine schools were undecided.[26] The American Council on Pharmaceutical Education issued its policy on accelerated programs at a March 27 meeting in which the decision of whether to accelerate was left up to the individual colleges. For those colleges that implemented an accelerated program the council suspended the requirement that two months elapse between academic years. From a student's perspective, a more important consideration was that those individuals (other than freshmen) who were inducted during the school year and who had completed more than half of the semester or quarter be allowed credit for the entire period if they could pass the necessary exams. The policy restated that any lessening of standards, including admissions, curriculum, or number of hours, would result in the loss of accreditation.[27]

NABP also accepted the need for acceleration and went on record that graduates of colleges which had implemented the three-year program would be eligible for reciprocity unless state law specifically prohibited it. In those states, boards were encouraged to get the legal interpretation necessary to facilitate reciprocity. The members of the boards believed that this would be fair to the students and colleges and minimize problems that might come up after the war.[28]

In 1943 Dean Rufus Lyman requested Dean Rudolph Kuever of the University of Iowa to do an early assessment of the accelerated program for publication in the *American Journal of Pharmaceutical Education*. Kuever reviewed the basis for the College of Pharmacy's decision to provide year-round courses. These included (1) the ability to complete the course in less time and (2) the increased number of students who could complete their education prior to going into the military. Kuever stated that the state Selective Service had indicated that as long as the students were in school continuously they would not draft students who had only one year, and in some cases two years, to complete their degree work. No slackening of quantity or quality of work was noted, and the college was operating on a forty-eight-week schedule. Costs associated with the pace of the accelerated program included longer days and few breaks. There were two weeks of vacation over the Christmas holidays and a one-week break between each of the other two semesters.[29]

The experience at Iowa was similar to that of other colleges of pharmacy that moved to the accelerated program. Charles Katsin recalls how the acceleration worked for him. He was one of the members of the entering class at Rutgers in 1940. When the college accelerated in 1942, students had to attend classes on Saturday and weekday class hours were lengthened. He received his call to report in April 1943 but was able to get a three-week delay so that he could get credit for the full semester before leaving school. His class graduated while he was in basic training at Newport, Rhode Island, and his diploma was mailed home.[30]

As if accelerating the four-year course into thirty-six months was not enough of a challenge, Louis B. Hershey, the director of Selective Service, raised the issue of an accelerated twenty-four-month program as a basis for occupational deferment for pharmacy students (see Chapter 3). At issue was the opportunity to defer students who would finish their educational program within twenty-four months of beginning it.[31] The general reaction from the colleges was that such a program would do grave harm to the advances that had been made in moving pharmacy to a baccalaureate degree requirement. Among others, Dean Robert C. Wilson of the University of Georgia expressed the position of his university that it was impossible to compress the accredited curriculum of 3,200 hours into a twenty-four-month program and under no circumstances would a BS degree be awarded for such an endeavor. Wilson also raised another issue, that of declining enrollments, by concluding, "It is our plan to continue to operate on the present accelerated basis (unsatisfactory as it is), and we hope to draw at least a sufficient number of students to justify the continuance of our program."[32]

The American Council on Pharmaceutical Education responded to the Selective Service's suggestion for a twenty-four-month program by developing conditions under which a college could maintain accreditation. Changed criteria included teaching load and size of classes, minimum admission requirements, and admission to advanced standing. For example, the maximum teaching load for faculty was set at twenty-four hours per week and the maximum number of students in a class should not exceed thirty. However, in spite of these changes, the curriculum remained at 3,200 contact hours, 1,300 of which were laboratory hours and had to include all of the required subjects listed in the fourth edition of the *Pharmaceutical Syllabus.* In his covering note, A. G. DuMez pointed out that the migration to any accelerated program, whether it was for twenty-four or thirty-six months, was at the option and discretion of the individual institution. The communication was intended to provide guidance to the institutions to maintain their accreditation. Buried in the note was the continuing recognition of enrollment shortages: "Some colleges may be able to secure a sufficient number of students from those under eighteen years of age, 4-Fs, and females to enable them to continue to operate as if conditions were normal."[33] Rutgers was a leader in moving to the superaccelerated program, and the colleges of pharmacy at the University of Maryland and Temple University were among the schools which announced the offering of a twenty-four-month program.[34]

There were vocal proponents of the superaccelerated program. In a letter to Charles H. Rogers, dean of the College of Pharmacy at the University of Minnesota and chair of the AACP Executive Committee, Robert Fischelis, then chair of the APhA Council, attached a note intended for the deans of the colleges of pharmacy that represented his thoughts regarding student deferments (whether this letter was ever sent to the deans is not known):

> I would accelerate my course to the utmost. This means getting the required 3200 hour course into twenty-four months of actual full time instruction. It can be done regardless of what you may think of it as an educational procedure. It is being done, and if you can't do it, you can expect no help by way of deferment of your students. This type of acceleration will automatically weed out weak students, and if you load up with poor quality materials you must expect a high mortality. Just as we demand the physically fit to fight at the front, so we must demand the mentally fit to carry on necessary professional services.[35]

At the 1943 AACP meeting a survey of the colleges was reported, in which only eight indicated their intention to adopt the superaccelerated twenty-four-month educational program while forty-one stated that they would not adopt such a shortened program. The AACP Executive Committee voted unanimously that the course leading to the BS in pharmacy "cannot be given in a period less than thirty-two-months of actual instruction"; this effectively blocked the offering of a twenty-four-month course.[36] Lee Adams, president of the National Association of the Boards of Pharmacy, reported that the boards supported this stance and declared that the thirty-two months of instruction (three-year program) was the minimum acceptable for registration by examination and reciprocity.[37,38] John Dargavel of NARD lauded the action of AACP and stated that "pharmacy as a profession has been guarded against the threat of lowering the standards as a measure, not of wartime necessity, but rather of wartime hysteria."[39] On October 6, 1943, ACPE rescinded its decision to allow accreditation for an accelerated program of less than thirty-two months. However, it allowed any school which had begun such a program to phase it out without negatively affecting students who had entered the courses in good faith.[40]

In response to the NABP position against the superacceleration programs and the rescinding of ACPE accreditation for the programs, there was a concern that students in those schools which had adopted the twenty-four-month program would either have to repeat some courses or would be refused the opportunity to take the state boards. The NABP Executive Committee addressed the situation in a bulletin to all boards and colleges on October 23, 1943. The recommendation of the committee was that since all of the colleges which implemented the twenty-four-month program were accredited and had acted in good faith, the students who would graduate in less than thirty-two months should not be disqualified for any time discrepancies. However, it was to be understood that all schools would discontinue the twenty-four-month program and return to a minimum of thirty-two months of instruction.[41]

AACP editor Rufus Lyman used his editorial page to discuss the tensions between ACPE and AACP as evidenced in the decision to accredit shortened courses and the rejection of offering them. Lyman's perspective was that the role of ACPE was to support the educational endeavor, not to force the accelerated programs, whether three or two year, on any of the colleges. Lyman felt that ACPE provided a buffer between the War Manpower Commission and the colleges. As the intermediary the council should facilitate the objectives of the commission in a way that would not diminish the quality of the educational program. Lyman believed that it was the responsibility of the individual colleges and AACP to decide whether to attempt an accelerated or even a superaccelerated program. He closed by stating that the personal criticisms of motive lodged against council representatives were not justified and that the attitude of the individual representatives toward both AACP and NABP was to be commended. [42]

Ernest Little, dean at the College of Pharmacy at Rutgers University and member of the ACPE, responded to Lyman's editorial and the discord. He challenged the concerns of whether pharmacy students were able to successfully complete a twenty-four-month course and calculated the hours necessary:

> If a student is in college from 9 o'clock until 12 o'clock and from 1 o'clock until 4 o'clock five days a week, and from 8 o'clock until noon on Saturday, he will, in a period of eight twelve-week terms covering a period of 24 months, have completed 3264 hours, which is in excess of the number of hours required for the Bachelor of Science in Pharmacy degree by either the AACP or the ACPE. Under this program, the student would have a schedule of 34 hours a week. He would have time for study late afternoons and evenings, five days a week. He would have Saturday afternoon and evening and all day Sunday available for study and recreation and would also have a full month of vacations during every calendar year.[43]

Little questioned whether this schedule was too heavy, given the nature of wartime, especially when medical students were carrying an excess of forty hours per week in their curriculum. His final point was that ACPE had merely allowed those colleges who wished to implement the superaccelerated program as a war measure to do so without losing accreditation.

In early 1944 the effectiveness of the three-year accelerated program was reviewed in the *American Journal of Pharmaceutical Education*. Charles H. Rogers, dean of the University of Minnesota College of Pharmacy, reviewed the assumptions for establishing the programs, which included the belief that military officials would demand properly trained pharmacy graduates as well as the need to provide replacements for civilian practice. The military demand never materialized; pharmacy technician programs were established instead. In addition, there was a perception that a significant pool of pharmacists could be drafted since so many were more involved in general merchandising than in the professional side of pharmacy. Rogers cited an example (unnamed) of a college that graduated seventy-two students in 1943; only seven women and one or two males who were 4-Fs were available for civilian employment. Rogers's conclusion was that the accelerated program had not met expectations and noted that the program at Minnesota would be discontinued with the fall 1944-1945 quarter.[44]

Some colleges also saw veterans returning to school before the end of the war. Some were men who were honorably discharged for a number of reasons, including permanent disabilities from wounds suffered in combat. For example, Ben Quintana was working as a hotel clerk and enlisted in the Marines immediately after Pearl Harbor. He was assigned to the First Marine Raiders and attached to the First Division. He took part in the action in the Guadal canal landings on August 7, 1942, and was wounded in action on September 13. After treatment he was discharged, and he enrolled in pharmacy at the University of Mississippi in 1943.[45]

In a private letter, Dean Christensen of the Ohio State University shared the school's experience of the accelerated program with J. G. Beard, dean of the college of pharmacy at the University of North Carolina. Christensen was favorably disposed to acceleration and believed that it had helped to increase enrollment, or at least lessen the decrease. He also felt that it was easier for students who failed a class to catch up since classes were repeated more often. Based on the experience of one year, the acceleration schedule was preferred to the prewar program, and Christensen reported considering continuing a year-round program after the war.[46]

The University of Minnesota undertook a study to compare the achievements of accelerated and nonaccelerated students, partly to determine whether any significant educational advances resulted from the shift. The comparative pools were relatively small and the measure limited to honor points of the two groups. The overall conclusion was that the students in the accelerated program did not score as well as their predecessors.[47]

At the 1944 AACP meeting C. O. Lee of the College of Pharmacy at Purdue University provided an evaluation of the accelerated program. In responding to a series of questions he noted that there was a lessening of standards and expectations, both for students and faculty, although the outcome was probably not bad. He concluded that the programs were a necessary response to the war emergency but had little to offer for normal times. Perhaps the most important observation was that the entire program was not designed to help students but to provide support for the military.[48]

Discontinuing the accelerated programs provided as many challenges as their implementation did. By 1944 at least forty-nine of the colleges were operating on an accelerated schedule; forty of these colleges were part of a university also operating on an accelerated schedule. The great unknown was the impact returning veterans would have on the course of study, especially in light of the recently passed Servicemen's Readjustment Act of 1944, better known as the GI Bill of Rights. Consequently, ACPE took the stance that it was impossible to set a definite date for the return to a four-year program and suggested that the recommendation to do so should come from the colleges themselves. [49]

WOMEN

In a review of the situation at the University of Michigan for the 1941-1942 academic year, Howard B. Lewis, director of the College of Pharmacy, reported that the total enrollment was slightly less than in the past, seventy-two compared to seventy-nine. He noted that the number of women remained relatively constant, and that in a period of increased demands from the military for registered pharmacists, the women graduates were "usefully employed."[50]

A number of colleges undertook recruiting programs to attract women to their schools in the hope of remaining open during the war. In a brochure titled, "Women in Science During the War and . . . After," the Philadelphia College of Pharmacy and Science told young women how they could be part of the war effort and the postwar period to follow. A reprinted editorial by Dean Ivor Griffith addressed

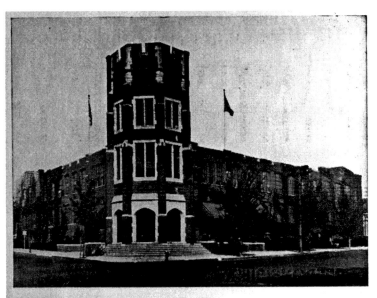

NEW JERSEY COLLEGE of PHARMACY, RUTGERS UNIVERSITY, NEWARK, N. J

The Woman Pharmacist

How many times have you heard the statement, "It doesn't matter too much what a young lady studies in college, because, following graduation, she will soon marry and devote most of her time to the important responsibility of homemaking." If that statement is true, how important it is that her college training should fit in as completely as possible with home duties. There can be few responsibilities as important as safeguarding the health of the family. The registered pharmacist's training is all centered around that important consideration.

The four-year course leading to the degree of Bachelor of Science in Pharmacy contains a reasonable number of cultural subjects, together with thorough training in the basic sciences such as chemistry, botany, zoology, bacteriology, elementary pathology, bio-chemistry, etc. The registered pharmacist of today must be a broadly educated person with a practical, specialized training which should prove of special value to the homemaker.

For further information, please address Miss Margaret Babbage, Registrar, Rutgers University, College of Pharmacy, 1 Lincoln Avenue, Newark 4, New Jersey. Telephone—HUmboldt 2-5670. Catalogues sent on request.

Colleges began to aggressively recruit women to increase enrollment. This ad is one of a series that the New Jersey College of Pharmacy developed for the state association journal. (*Source: New Jersey Journal of Pharmacy* [1944] 17: cover 2. Photo courtesy of the Lloyd Library and Museum. Reprinted with permission.)

the dramatis personae, that is, "the Old Fogeys and Fuss-pots of the Medical Society on the proposed establishment of the *Female* Medical College in Philadelphia," and used the opportunity to talk about women pharmacists. After reviewing the history of women in pharmacy in Philadelphia, he concluded by noting that the scholastic performance of women was equal to that of their male counterparts and that many had earned professional honors.[51] Yet before World War II the numbers of women in pharmacy were few. For example, the 1940 census reported 4 percent of pharmacists were women; according to AACP 12 percent of the students in 1940-1941 were women.[52]

The New Jersey College of Pharmacy of Rutgers University ran a series of advertisements in the *New Jersey Journal of Pharmacy* that were addressed to women. In one advertisement the college explained how the education of a pharmacist would help a woman with her duties as a housewife:

> How many times have you heard the statement, "It doesn't matter too much what a young lady studies in college, because, following graduation, she will soon marry and devote most of her time to the important responsibility of homemaking." If that statement is true, how important it is that her college training should fit in as completely as possible with home duties. There can be few responsibilities as important as safeguarding the health of the family. The registered pharmacist's training is all centered around that important consideration.[53]

In another advertisement the college addressed the topic of "Your Daughter's Education" and encouraged fathers to suggest that their daughters contact Rutgers University College of Pharmacy.[54]

A similar recruiting effort was undertaken by a number of pharmacy associations and groups. The Oregon State Pharmaceutical Association distributed a pamphlet to the high school graduating class of 1943. The pamphlet asked and answered a series of questions about career opportunities, differences in salaries between men and women, and helping the war effort. Interested women were invited to contact the School of Pharmacy at the state university.[55]

Lois Hummel Nekrassoff provided a perspective of her education in a college with few students and the length to which schools went to stay viable. She enrolled at the University of Tennessee after a year of prepharmacy at the then–University of Chattanooga. The program was operated twelve months a year with two weeks off at Christmas and another two in June. The students had the option to add an eighteen-month medical technology program to their pharmacy studies at no additional cost. The College of Pharmacy combined some classes with the dental and medical schools since those students were deferred or in one of the military training programs. During her junior and senior years there were only about fifteen students in the entire college and the graduation class was made up of four women and two men.[56]

A 1944 editorial in *Pacific Drug Review* reported that recruiting efforts had been successful. In one school in the Pacific Northwest (otherwise unidentified) twenty-six of the thirty entering students and two-thirds of the student body were women. Other schools reported that women made up between one-third and one-half of the student body. However, the increase in women did not make up for the loss of men, since enrollments in the schools had decreased by over 50 percent. The conclusion was that the schools would not have been able to continue to operate without an increase in the enrollment of women. The overall situation was put into a practice picture by stating the entire graduating classes in all six schools of the Pacific Slope would number only seventy-two, and that in an area with approximately 6,000 drugstores.[57]

JAPANESE AMERICANS

In May 1942, the College of Pharmacy at the University of California noted that Japanese American students had been forced to leave school by the Western Defense Command of the Army.[58] In October, Forest J. Goodrich of the College of Pharmacy at the University of Washington reported that all twenty-six Japanese American students had been removed and for the first time in many years there would be none present when school opened for the fall term.[59] The University of Southern California reported in November that there was no one of Japanese descent enrolled because all of them had been removed from the Pacific Coast.[60] In 1941 there were at least 3,252 college students of Japanese ancestry attending schools in California, Oregon, and Washington; in 1943 there were sixty.[61] While these reports labeled the students as Japanese, they were really American-born citizens of Japanese ancestry; the authorities were not open about admitting the removal of rights from citizens.

The Asian immigrant population of the West Coast had never assimilated well, due in part to laws that precluded those born in Japan from ever achieving American citizenship. However, their children, the Nisei generation, were American-born citizens. On February 19, 1942, President Roosevelt signed Executive Order 9066 establishing military zones and authorizing the military commander to exclude any individual at his discretion.[62] This order forced over 110,000 people from their homes, schools, and businesses into ten hastily constructed relocation camps in Idaho (Minidoka), Arizona (Colorado River, Gila River), Arkansas (Rohwer, Jerome), Colorado (Granada), Wyoming (Heart Mountain), Utah (Central Utah), and eastern California (Tule Lake, Manzanar).

Pharmacy students were removed from classes at the University of Washington, Oregon State College, University of California, and the University of Southern California. The options available were to go to the camps with their families or to find another pharmacy school outside of the exclusion zone that would accept them. Neither class standing nor citizenship was sufficient to keep the students in their original schools. Kiyo Fuji, Toshio Noma, and Mary Shimoda were among the ten students admitted to Rho Chi at the University of Washington in the spring of 1942.[63] In one documented case, Dean Troy Daniels at the University of California College of Pharmacy offered, unsuccessfully, to adopt a Nisei graduate student, Harry Iwamoto, so that he could stay in school and finish his degree.[64]

The number of pharmacy students affected is unknown. It was impossible to identify any pharmacy students among the 3,530 Nisei students in a 1941 national survey. Certainly there were no Nisei students identified at the independent pharmacy schools, such as the St. Louis College of Pharmacy or Philadelphia College of Pharmacy. The 1943 survey reported twelve Nisei students at the St. Louis College of Pharmacy.[65] A number of students were allowed to transfer to pharmacy schools at the University of Idaho Southern Branch and the University of Nebraska. Victoria Dickinson enrolled in the College of

Pharmacy at the University of Nebraska in 1942; her class had thirty men and three women, but by 1943 all of the men had been drafted. She recalled that the college enrolled five displaced Japanese students. "My memory of them is one of young men who were determined to achieve. I cannot remember a single instance of complaint as to why they were there—I only know I had to work hard to keep up."[66] Eugene Tatsuru Kimura was accepted at the University of Nebraska from the Assembly Center in Puyallup, Washington, and graduated in 1944. He recalled that he was "fortunate to have been accepted as a student. Students and faculty were friendly, understanding and helpful. Only a few townspeople were bigoted and unfriendly." His brother, Kazuo Kimura, also transferred and later acknowledged the helpfulness of Rufus Lyman.[67]

POSTWAR PLANNING

In the midst of dealing with the draft and accelerated classes, the questions of postwar problems and opportunities were on the table. During the NABP/AACP District 1 meeting in March 1943, Leslie Barrett of the University of Connecticut proposed a list of issues that included the resumption of a normal four-year educational cycle and the need to deal with granting college credit for military experience, especially that gained through the pharmacy technician program.[68] By the end of the year the AACP's Committee on Long Range Program of Policy developed a list of assumptions for the postwar period along with a lengthy list of objectives which included the maintenance of educational standards and the prevention of excessive numbers of pharmacy graduates.[69]

By 1944, as Congress was considering what types of subsidies to award to those who had served in the military, AACP leadership began to plan for the postwar period. The military had started discharging veterans at the rate of 90,000 per month, some of whom were ready to finish the education that had been delayed by military service. Bernard V. Christensen, dean of the College of Pharmacy at Ohio State University, laid out the challenges that professional education was likely to face in the immediate postwar period. He first reviewed the background that pharmacy practice was governed by state laws and that all states required graduation from an accredited college. As a corollary, he emphasized that the military's pharmacy technician programs did not meet accreditation standards. He went on to summarize three needs: (1) educational programs at the professional, sub- or preprofessional, postgraduate, and refresher program levels; (2) facilities and qualified teaching personnel; and, (3) funding.[70] An editorial by Dean H. C. Newton in the same issue of the *American Journal of Pharmaceutical Education* divided the students-to-be into four groups. The first was a group of approximately 1,500 who had planned on entering pharmacy school but went into the military instead. The second group was individuals who might decide on pharmacy as a career as a consequence of their military service. The third and potentially largest group consisted of those individuals who withdrew from pharmacy school for military service. The number was estimated in the thousands. The fourth group was pharmacists who had been away from practice during their military service and were looking for a refresher course before reentering practice.[71]

In 1944 Forest J. Goodrich, University of Washington College of Pharmacy and AACP president, appointed a committee to consider postwar planning. In an attempt to evolve a broad perspective the committee solicited input from each member college of AACP. The committee posed thirteen questions that covered a broad scope, ranging from the fate of the accelerated programs and the treatment of returning students, to the status quo of the curricula and the prepharmacy year requirement. The committee received forty-five responses, including one from the National Association of Boards of Pharmacy. As might be expected, there were many points of view and there was little consensus.[72]

In its report to AACP, the committee agreed unanimously on discontinuing the accelerated three-year program but was not willing to set a definite date for implementation. Again, the GI Bill was an unknown determinant. The committee recognized that many veterans went into the service before finishing high school and would probably seek early college admission. The committee recommended that admission standards for such students not be lowered under any circumstances. The questions relating to the change and development of a professional curriculum, coordination of the curriculum with other health professions, and the role of the profession were left for later discussion and decision.[73]

AMERICAN FOUNDATION
FOR PHARMACEUTICAL EDUCATION

In August 1942 the American Foundation for Pharmaceutical Education was incorporated by representatives of nine organizations. These were the American Association of Colleges of Pharmacy, American Drug Manufacturers Association, American Pharmaceutical Association, American Pharmaceutical Manufacturers Association, Federal Wholesale Druggists' Association, National Association of Boards of Pharmacy, National Association of Retail Druggists, National Wholesale Druggists' Association, and Proprietary Association. The National Association of Chain Drug Stores formally joined the foundation in 1943.* The foundation was created by combining the Committee on Endowment of the National Drug Trade Conference and the All Industry Scholarship Committee of the National Wholesale Druggists' Association into one entity.[74] The formation of the foundation was in direct response to the growing need for financial support both for individual students and for colleges. The purpose of the foundation was to collect and administer funds to aid and strengthen pharmacy education. In the report of the formation of the foundation to the American Association of Colleges of Pharmacy, Ernest Little stated four objectives:

1. Help worthy colleges to develop strong undergraduate programs. This obligation might very properly be considered as the foundation's major responsibility;
2. Support graduate work in colleges which they deem qualified to carry on such programs in a creditable manner;

---

*By 2003 seven of the nine associations had changed their names. The American Drug Manufacturers Association and the American Pharmaceutical Manufacturers Association merged into the Pharmaceutical Manufacturers Association in 1958 and was renamed the Pharmaceutical Research and Manufacturers of America in 1994. The National Association of Retail Druggists moved to the use of the acronym NARD and in 1996 changed its name to the National Community Pharmacists Association. The Federal Wholesale Druggists' Association merged with the National Wholesale Druggists' Association (NWDA) in 1984; in 2001, NWDA changed its name to the Healthcare Distribution Management Association. The Proprietary Association changed its name to the Nonprescription Drug Manufacturers Association in 1990 and, in 1999, to Consumer Health Care Products Association. The American Pharmaceutical Association changed its name to the American Pharmacists Association in 2003.

3. Encourage scientific research, both as a necessary component of graduate work and as special projects; and,

4. Render such general and special help as they consider wise and appropriate, such as the maintenance of scholarship and loan funds for worthy students and the promotion of other projects too numerous to be mentioned individually.[75]

The first priority of the foundation was to strengthen the undergraduate professional programs, helping those colleges which had suffered most in enrollment decreases. While there was a willingness to consider graduate education, that would have to come later when the funds were available and schools were capable of providing high-quality programs.

AFPE immediately undertook two separate surveys to determine the financial status of the colleges of pharmacy. The findings showed that seventeen of the sixty-four colleges had deficits totaling more than $200,000, and some faced the possibility of closing without outside financial aid. In May 1944 the foundation authorized up to $62,000 in emergency war aid to the thirteen schools which had the most pressing needs (see Table 2.4).[76] In reporting these grants, Edward Rogers, chair of the foundation's Grants Committee, reaffirmed that the foundation's long-range goals were to support scholarships for professional education, provide temporary grants to colleges to keep them operating, and develop fellowships to strengthen the faculties.[77] In December 1943, the foundation provided two $200 scholarships to each of the sixty-four accredited colleges, thus providing approximately 128 scholarships for pharmacy students. In 1944 the foundation continued the 1943 distribution of two $200 scholarships to the accredited colleges of pharmacy and in 1945 allocated $100 for scholarship at each college. [78,79]

A few educators had concerns over the makeup of the foundation, fearing that the financial interests of the wholesalers and manufacturers might conflict with the professional idealism of education. Rufus Lyman, after attending the initial meeting between the executive council of AACP and the board of AFPE, challenged such thinking, stating:

We make a great mistake if we in our thinking arrive at the conclusion that all of the idealism in pharmacy is centered in the educational group. Men in industry have quite as much idealism and what is most important in matters educational they are willing to be led by the educational group. What they will expect, and rightfully, is that any funds allotted to pharmaceutical education be used wisely and show objectives accomplished.[80]

TABLE 2.4. American Foundation for Pharmaceutical Education Emergency War Aid, 1944

College	Amount of Cash Grant	Conditions
Albany College of Pharmacy	$4,500	
Brooklyn College of Pharmacy	$7,500	
Cincinnati College of Pharmacy	$5,000	Agreement to match up to $2,000 from funds raised locally
Creighton University	$3,000	Conditional on matching funds raised locally
Duquesne College of Pharmacy	$3,500	
Ferris Institute	$3,000	
Louisville College of Pharmacy	$2,500	Agreement to match up to $2,000 from funds raised locally
New York College of Pharmacy (later called Columbia)	$5,000	
Philadelphia College of Pharmacy	$7,500	
Southern College of Pharmacy	$3,500	Agreement to match up to $1,500 from funds raised locally
Western Reserve University	$4,500	Conditional on matching funds raised locally
Xavier University	$3,000	
St. Louis College of Pharmacy	$4,000	

Source: Fisher, A. B. (1992). *A Half Century of Service to Pharmacy, 1942-1992.* Rockville, MD: The American Foundation for Pharmaceutical Education, pp. 1-2.

A difference of opinion occurred between the AACP representatives and those of the foundation on how the scholarship funds should be awarded. The stance of AACP was that the scholarships should be reserved for the top scholastic students, while AFPE opted for the students in most need of financial support.[81] In the end, the minimum requirements for a scholarship were based on the student's need of financial support and (1) a high school graduate in the upper fiftieth percentile of the class or (2) a college student with proven competency and ability with a minimum of a C average. The selection of the winners was left to the discretion of the individual colleges, as was the duration of the scholarship. The only conditions required by AFPE were that the colleges report (1) the name of the recipient and the basis for selection and (2) the grades earned while receiving the scholarship. In addition, the scholarship funds were to be restricted to use for tuition, fees, and books.[82]

STUDENT FINANCES

University professional and scientific educational programs which adopted accelerated schedules claimed that students faced financial hardships largely due to the inability to take summer jobs. AACP convinced the U.S. Office of Education of the shortage of pharmacists and the need to accelerate the four-year program to three to address the shortage. Thus, pharmacy was added to the list of professions to be considered for federal aid, along with engineering, physics, chemistry, medicine, veterinary medicine, and dentistry. [83]

The Office of Education gained funds for student loans but was unable to gain similar aid for the educational institutions. The appropriation act was passed in June 1942 as "Provisions for Loans to Students in Certain Accelerated Programs." The conditions for these loans were that the students would complete their education within a twenty-four-month period and maintain a satisfactory level of scholarship. In addition, the students had to agree to accept the employment or service assigned by the chairman of the War Manpower Commission. Loans were restricted to tuition and fees along with a stipend of twenty-five dollars per month; the total could not exceed $500 per year. The loans carried an interest rate of 2.5 percent per year. In the event that the student was drafted before completing the program, the loan was canceled. Similarly, if the student was killed or disabled in the military, the debt was canceled.[84] During the first year of the program, ending June 30, 1943, 438 pharmacy students from sixty-seven colleges received loans under the program. The average loan was $257 per student. The program was scaled back in fiscal 1944, and loans became limited to students who had received loans the previous year.[85]

Finances for many colleges remained a problem throughout the war years. This was especially true for the private schools that depended largely on tuition as the main source of income. The Cincinnati College of Pharmacy was a good example of the problem. In the prewar period the average student body was about 250 students, but by the summer of 1945 the total enrollment was thirty-six.[86] Low enrollment continued until the 1945-1946 academic year when the release of large numbers from the military increased college enrollment.

REFRESHER COURSES

Refresher courses for the men who had served in the military were considered a postwar need. Many veterans had not practiced pharmacy at all during their service time. Those who did had worked in an environment much different from what they would encounter in postwar civilian practice.

In 1944, Bernard V. Christensen of Ohio State suggested that the postwar refresher course last three to four and one-half months. He thought that the participants would need a survey course covering all branches of pharmacy education, including pharmaceutical chemistry, pharmacognosy, and pharmacology. The course would also bring the returning veterans up to date on the advances and new products.[87] Rufus Lyman took a different position, stating that few returning veterans would be interested in taking a cram course but, instead, would opt to get back into a routine just as quickly as possible. He thought that a course of less than a week's duration to cover new developments would be about as much as could be expected.[88] Thomas Rowe of the Medical College of Virginia reviewed the options that had been discussed and clearly preferred the shorter period over the longer, based on the likely reality of time and money that a veteran was willing to spend. Rowe suggested four topics that should be covered in any refresher program: two of the topics were a general review of pharmacy (including dispensing) and new trends, such as product prices, availability, and legal restrictions. Another topic was devoted to new developments—both technical and legal—and the final topic covered laboratory technique, such as the manufacture of dose forms including suppositories and powders.[89]

CREDIT FOR MILITARY SERVICE

On June 9, 1942, Charles H. Rogers, chair of the Executive Committee of AACP, wrote to Surgeon General of the Army James C. Magee requesting a statement that the Army's pharmacy technician program did not in any way qualify individuals to either take a state board examination or practice pharmacy. Concern grew on the part of many pharmacy leaders that the refusal of the Army to assign only registered pharmacists to pharmaceutical duties and the expansion of the pharmacy technician programs would lead postwar veterans to claim that their military service was sufficient experience to be licensed. Magee's response, as reported to the AACP's membership, was considered to clearly represent the military's position on the question:

> It is difficult to understand how this type of abbreviated and carefully planned training to meet the urgent needs of the Medical Department could contribute to the lowering of the established standards of pharmaceutical education formulated by the American Pharmaceutical Association or other related agencies. It is equally difficult to see how these methods of meeting temporary requirements of the Army should in any way influence the standards of licensure now established. The purpose of the enlisted technicians' schools was and is still to meet the temporary and urgent requirements for an auxiliary service to the Medical Department—a need created first by the tempo of mobilization and extended later by the urgency of war, and not to lower the educational requirements of any civilian institution or licensure standards now established.[90]

The issue of academic credit for military experience was larger than just the pharmacy technicians program. Many young men attended college-level courses through one of the military's training programs, such as the Navy V-12. In these programs individuals were assigned to programs on a college campus that would either prepare them for a specific assignment, such as signals officer, or as a preparation for a commissioned officer's training program. Many others in the Armed Forces took correspondence courses, either on their own or as part of a military program. The AACP's Committee on Educational and Membership Standards was one of the first to look at the question of accrediting various experiences in the military; NABP and ACPE were also interested. The committee recommended that any accreditation be limited to instances in which the military activity corresponded closely with its civilian counterpart. The committee also recommended that any college-level work be assessed for content and quality as well as clock-hour equivalence and suggested that competency tests be considered in scientific subjects. The committee also recommended that any blanket accreditation for military service be prohibited.[91]

In October 1943, the American Council on Pharmaceutical Education appointed a special committee charged with developing guidelines for accreditation of military experience.[92] In April 1944, the American Association of Colleges of Pharmacy and the National Association of Boards of Pharmacy formed a joint committee to examine the same issues.[93] ACPE offered recommendations on the treatment of educational experiences in the military to its sponsoring organizations (AACP, NABP, and APhA) during its 1944 annual meeting. The recommendations included the following:

1. It is recommended that colleges of pharmacy give no credit for work experiences such as employment in military hospital dispensaries, even if done in well regulated hospitals. In the opinion of the committee, credit for this kind of work might more appropriately be given by boards of pharmacy toward the practical experience requirement for licensure.
2. It is recommended that any credit extended be granted on the basis of educational values received, rather than courses taken or experience gained. This means careful testing, usually by means of formal examinations of many of the applicants applying for college credit.
3. It is recommended that the policy of the colleges should be to extend appropriate but conservative college credit for military

activities. The committee suggests that the maximum amount of credit allowed for military activities of all sorts should usually be less than one-eighth of the requirements for the B.S. degree. Credit should be allowed only for such subjects as may be considered fully equivalent to the same or similar subjects in the degree course and never in excess of an hour for hour basis.

4. The granting of blanket credit for military experience is strongly advised against, except as a basic military training and indoctrination program required for all men and women in the armed forces may be credit toward the colleges' military training, physical education, first-aid or hygiene requirement. Credits, so permitted, should be conservatively granted and never in excess of the amount of such work required or permitted by the college for the degree under consideration.[94]

In 1945, Robert Fischelis, the APhA secretary, addressed the issue of granting credit for military experience during a speech at the University of Buffalo College of Pharmacy. He noted that the veteran should be allowed reasonable credit for military experience but not at the cost of relaxing the necessary requirements. The individual whose education or training was interrupted by military service should be given every chance to complete the requirements for obtaining his license as a registered pharmacist. However, doing something for the individual that would erode professional standards would help neither the individual nor the public.[95]

Chapter 3

Selective Service

Manpower, or the lack of it, was one of the most pervasive and persistent issues in the United States during World War II. Manpower issues also affected pharmacy—especially education and retail. The war opened the debate over whether there were shortages of pharmacists and whether these shortages were national or local. The discussion expanded to what the root causes of any shortages were, including the inappropriate employment of registered pharmacists in civilian life. The debate also embroiled the military as men were drafted from pharmacies to serve not as pharmacists but in many different assignments, including infantry and artillery. Consequently, manpower utilization, rather than just numerical availability, became the common issue that eddied between the military and the profession.

THE SELECTIVE TRAINING
AND SERVICE ACT OF 1940

On September 16, 1940, the Burke-Wadsworth Bill passed Congress and became Public Law 783 as the Selective Training and Service Act of 1940.[1] One month later, the registration period for all males between the ages of twenty-one to thirty-six began, and thirteen days later, on October 29, 1940, Secretary of War Stimson drew the capsule containing the first number of the draft lottery.[2] Those drafted were to serve in the active forces for twelve consecutive months and in the reserve for ten additional years or until the age of forty-five. In the event that Congress declared it necessary for national defense, the active-duty period could be extended and the reserves called to active duty.

The act established the Selective Service system; federal employees or the military staffed the national and state offices. National headquarters had the responsibility to set policy and determine the number of men required to meet the needs of the military. The quotas were broken down to state levels and then further broken down for the local boards to fill. Volunteers staffed the more than 6,000 local boards.[3] One of the lessons learned during the Civil War and implemented in World War I was the need for a local voice in the selection of who would be drafted and who would remain in the community. Thus, the final choice of who would be called or deferred rested with local boards.

The act also established deferment for men whose employment was necessary for the maintenance of the national health, safety, or interest. While the national headquarters developed the criteria for a "necessary man," it was up to the local boards to decide who the necessary men were. The act also established that any deferment should be made on a case-by-case basis and thus proscribed deferment of any occupational group or groups at any plant or institution.

PRE–PEARL HARBOR

Pharmacists and pharmacy students were among those drafted in the early months of 1941. Common questions were whether students could be deferred to complete their education and whether pharmacists were, by definition, necessary men. Once drafted, the questions focused on whether pharmacists would be commissioned as officers and how to gain an assignment as a pharmacist. Each of these questions would continue to be raised throughout the course of the war.

Students could ask for an educational deferment if they were drafted in the early months of conscription. The original act provided for a group deferment for all full-time students at colleges and universities until the end of the academic year but no later than July 1, 1941. Any extension of a student's deferment was left to the individual's draft board; the criteria used by the board was whether the student was being trained in a field or discipline necessary for the country's welfare.

Pharmacists were not automatically deferred as necessary men. The decision of who was or was not a necessary man was made by each man's draft board. While pharmaceutical services were generally considered necessary for the maintenance of health and safety of the civilian population, it was up to the local draft board to determine whether an individual pharmacist was necessary to the health and welfare of his community. The issue of being "necessary to the community" was an important criterion, as draft boards and the profession tried to sort through the mix of services that a pharmacist provided, i.e., whether the professional pharmaceutical services outweighed the provision of other services and goods, such as proprietary products, candy, tobacco, and fountain service.

Pharmacists were not commissioned to provide pharmaceutical services in the military. The armed forces had a long history of regarding pharmacists as shopkeepers and technicians and so had resisted establishing a commissioned corps for pharmacists (see Chapter 6). Pharmacists were eligible to apply for a commission in the Medical Administrative Corps of the Army. The applicant had to meet all of the requirements of the Army, including education, leadership ability, and the subjective requirement of being "officer material." However, pharmacists who were commissioned in the Medical Administrative Corps would not be filling prescriptions and might even have no duties associated with pharmacy. Pharmacists who were drafted also had the opportunity to apply for Officer's Candidate School and, if successfully commissioned, serve in any area of the Army.

Pharmacists were advised to identify themselves as such and ask to be placed in pharmaceutical duties. They were warned, however, that the Army could assign them to any duty, based on the needs of the service. Assignments would be based on a number of factors, including the qualifications of the individual involved. This was an important consideration because a majority of pharmacists did not have a four-year college degree. The mandatory bachelor's degree was not universally implemented until 1932, and a significant number of draft-age pharmacists had only a two- or three-year pharmacy degree.[4]

H. Evert Kendig, chair of the Committee on the Status of Pharmacists in the Government Service, emphasized that all of the judgments of the Selective Service process were based on the individual, not the group or class:

> No group, class, or profession receives a blanket consideration. Pharmacists as a class are not exempt, or deferred. Pharmacists, as a class, are not assured of commissions. Pharmacists, as a class, are not even assured that they will be placed in positions where they will perform pharmaceutical duties. It is the individual, his civilian circumstances, and both his educational and general qualifications, as well as the requirements of the Army, which must be considered.[5]

In August 1941, Francis J. Brown, a representative of the American Council on Education, spoke on Selective Service student deferments in general and for pharmacy students in particular. He outlined the creation of the National Committee on Education and Defense and its Subcommittee on Military Affairs. The subcommittee was invited by the Selective Service system to develop a list of professions that were necessary for national defense. A number of basic sciences, such as chemistry and physics, as well as medicine, dentistry, and pharmacy were included. He noted that medical students were almost universally deferred, including those individuals who had completed undergraduate work and were awaiting admission to a medical school. However, he continued, pharmacy was not as successful in gaining student deferments and suggested that the problem was due in part to a divergence in opinion concerning pharmacist shortages by pharmacy leadership itself. Some leaders, he noted, "believe that there are too many service station drugstores hence too many pharmacists. Others equally sincere believe there was an actual and growing acute shortage."[6]

MANPOWER

The issue of pharmacy manpower shortages had two components. The first component was practitioners; the second was students. The broadest issue was the shortage of licensed pharmacists in practice, predominantly in retail settings. While student shortages created problems for the colleges (see Chapter 2), it was the lack of new practitioners that gained the attention of the entire profession.

In 1941, there was disagreement about whether a shortage of pharmacists existed. In a 1941 editorial in the *American Journal of Pharmaceutical Education,* Rufus Lyman spoke out against the presumed shortage of pharmacists and noted that there were many towns in his home state of Nebraska that would be better served with fewer drugstores. Some believed a shortage existed as a consequence of fewer graduations—due first to the mandated transition from a three- to a four-year course of study in the 1930s and second to the residual effect of the Depression—and that the draft exacerbated the shortage. Others believed there was no real shortage of pharmacists doing professional work; any perception of shortage was due to the nonprofessional activities of the pharmacist. An unsigned editorial most likely written by Robert Fischelis in the *New Jersey Journal of Pharmacy* under the heading "The Shortage (?) of Pharmacists" took the position that there was no shortage:

> The facts are that there is little or no shortage of pharmacists anywhere in the United States today. Anyone looking the situation squarely in the face and without any axe to grind would have to admit that one-half the number of pharmacies now in existence could supply all legitimate pharmaceutical services needed by the people of the United States and still leave an over-supply of such service.[7]

R. A. Kuever, dean of the College of Pharmacy at the University of Iowa, described some pharmacy averages in an opinion article. He noted a national average of one drugstore for each 2,000 people; the average family spent between twenty and twenty-five dollars per year for medicines. According to Kuever there were 57,000 drugstores filling 250,000,000 prescriptions per year; however, these prescriptions accounted for only 10 percent of the dollar volume. Using these figures, an average drugstore filled less than twelve prescriptions per day in a 365-day year. The remaining 90 percent of the store's business was dependent on the "resourcefulness of the pharmacist and his ability at merchandising."[8] In fact, the Office of Production Management had not found a national shortage of pharmacists prior to the outbreak of hostilities. In some local situations shortages occurred, and they were addressed by local draft boards.[9] An underlying com-

ponent of the manpower shortage was that state laws required a registered pharmacist to be on duty when the drugstore was open, no matter how many prescriptions were actually presented or filled.

In 1942 the Bureau of Census released a report on occupational
employment based on the 1940 census. The report provided a snapshot of the manpower situation as it existed during the week of March
23-30, prior to the start of the war. The census showed 81,924 available practitioners. This was almost 25 percent less than the aggregate
total taken from state boards' total of 107,322—which included a
number of pharmacists who were registered in more than one state
and were consequently counted more than once, as well as pharmacists no longer in practice. The potential manpower shortfall was calculated by using the actuarial replacement figure of 2.6 percent per
year for personnel losses due to death or retirement. Consequently,
2,126 newly licensed pharmacists were needed each year just to
maintain the 1940 manpower level, which many considered far too
low. In 1940 only 1,511 students graduated from the colleges of pharmacy; between the years of 1941 and 1945 fewer than 9,000 students
graduated. This figure was likely understated since it included reports
only from those colleges who were members of the American Association of the Colleges of Pharmacy. According to the census, the
gender composition of the profession was 78,708 men (96 percent)
and 3,216 women (4 percent). Of the total number of students 7,945
(88 percent) were men. The census also reported 57,903 drugstores in
operation in 1939.[10,11] These data would provide the basis for pharmacy's argument for student deferment and "necessary men" classification for the entire war period.

The Selective Service issued Memorandum I-405 and Local Board
Release 115 in March, 1942. The memorandum's subject was occupational classification; it opened with the statement that the advisory
was to be referred to frequently in future considerations of occupational classification. The advisory clearly defined the balance that Selective Service needed to achieve:

> The Selective Service System has the responsibility to select
> men for military service and to furnish them at the time and in
> the number necessary for the Armed Forces of the nation. On
> the other hand, the Selective Service System has the corollary

responsibility to select for retention in their civilian endeavor an adequate supply of trained, qualified, or skilled men in order to maintain those civilian activities necessary to war production and other civilian activities essential to the support of the war effort.

Part III of the Memorandum addressed "Civilian Activities Supporting the War Effort." War production was clearly the most important classification; all other categories addressed supporting that effort. What constituted necessary was clearly stated.

Now that we are at war the phrase "national health, safety, or interest" *no longer includes mere convenience and comfort.* Activities essential to the national health, safety or interest are now linked to those activities, other than war production, which supports the war effort. Activities supporting the war effort include those activities which provide food, clothing, shelter, health, safety, and other requisites of our daily life. (emphasis added)[12]

In January 1943 the state advisor on occupational deferments wrote to the Minnesota pharmacy association concerning the ongoing deferments of both pharmacists and pharmacy students. The official noted that Selective Service had been responsive to the requests for deferment but called the attention of the association to changes in occupational requirements for deferment. He noted that pharmacists, engaged in the practice of pharmacy, could be considered for deferment but noted that it was important to consider the amount of time spent in filling prescriptions as part of the deferment criteria. An example was given of a two-man store where much of the pharmacists' time was spent in merchandising and sales activities rather than filling prescriptions. In such cases, it would be appropriate to defer one pharmacist who could take on the entire dispensing role while drafting the other.[13]

The lack of an accurate census of pharmacists continued to hamper arguments for deferment of pharmacists. In an attempt to improve on the 1940 census, Fischelis and George Fiero published a quantitative report on the civilian needs for pharmacists in 1943. They reported a total of 70,449 pharmacists available for retail practice. Civilian requirements, based on the number of pharmacies, the size of community, and prescription volume, were 65,680 pharmacists. The military expected that 12,240 pharmacists would be taken into the Armed Forces. This meant that there would be an estimated shortage of 7,471 pharmacists, with a consequential closure of 6,500 pharmacies.[14] One concern was the inability to provide a consistent level of pharmacy service in all locales: stores could not be moved, and the draft was uncertain and inconsistent from one community to another, much less from one state to another. As late as 1944 some Selective Service officials discussed the possibility of closing pharmacies and centralizing all prescription services into the remaining stores.[15] In New York State the Selective Service director noted that the only reason there was a shortage was because of the requirement to have a pharmacist on duty in a drugstore whenever it was open. Since filling prescriptions took only a small fraction of the pharmacist's professional time, he indicated that centralization was a possible solution.[16]

In 1943 the Bureau of Business Research of Ohio State University, in cooperation with the State Board and Association, undertook a comprehensive pharmacy manpower study. The purpose was to provide accurate documentation on manpower rather than to prove a shortage existed. The data were available to all groups as they worked toward developing a balance between military and civilian needs. The Ohio Manpower Study provided detailed information on the number of pharmacists, their gender, and draft classifications at the city and county level. There were 4,768 pharmacists in Ohio, 4,506 males and 262 females. The only race information given is for white and "colored." Of the forty colored pharmacists in the state, thirty-five were male and five female. Eighty-eight percent of all pharmacists worked in retail pharmacy. Most pharmacists had three years of college education or less and approximately only 20 percent had a BS degree. These data were valuable in answering questions of shortages and distribution for the profession, as well as the State Selective Service and local draft boards.

The Ohio Manpower study data also provided a trenchant insight into the use of the 320 Ohio pharmacists already in the military. To the question of whether these individuals were performing pharmaceutical services, of those responding, 49 percent indicated that they were not.[17]

STUDENTS AND THE COLLEGES

In March 1941 Selective Service issued Memorandum I-10 to state directors identifying the accurate classification of students training in essential professions as one of its major problems.[18] In April, Selective Service released Memorandum I-62 to state directors advising them that students who were in training or preparation for occupations necessary for national health and safety should be deferred. Suggested considerations of appropriate student classification were the length of time that the students had been in training, their progress and achievement in the course, and their chances of employment. The deferment was to be given for only six months but could be renewed. The advisory concluded with the admonition that such deferments were to be considered on an individual basis and should not be granted to whole groups. In a subsequent advisory to state directors, engineering and chemistry were identified as fields having a dangerously low level of civilian manpower. A second list of professions, including dentistry, medicine, and pharmacy, was identified as occupations where "authorities allege that a shortage will exist, but which have not yet been studied."[19]

The 1942 Selective Service Memorandum I-405 and Local Board Release 115 provided local boards with considerable guidance on what constituted a "necessary man in training." These publications set standards that would be applied to pharmacy students who were seeking opportunities for education-based deferment. Apprentices and others who were being trained on the job were not considered to be in training, since their classification as a necessary man could be determined by the work in which they were engaged. There was a tacit recognition that it was easier to identify those in training for a particular occupation, such as a welder. It was more difficult to determine whether those in academic programs were in training for an essential occupation. Consequently, it was suggested that satisfactory work through at least two years of academic training was required before classifying a student as a necessary man in training. At that point the man must continue to meet all of the criteria, plus the occupation must continue to be considered essential to the war effort. Selective Service established four conditions, and all must be met to be considered for deferment as a necessary man in training:

(a) He must be in training to acquire a qualification or skill which fits him for a "critical occupation" in an activity necessary to war production or essential to the support of the war effort;

(b) There must be an existing or contemplated shortage of persons, in activities necessary to war production or essential to the support of the war effort, who possess the training, qualification or skill which the registrant is in training and preparation to acquire;

(c) There must be a shortage of persons who are undertaking such training and preparation to the extent that even though all such persons successfully complete the training and preparation and enter "critical occupations" in activities necessary to war production or essential to the support of the war effort, the shortage existing in those activities will not be entirely relieved; and,

(d) He must have advanced sufficiently in his training and preparation that there is a reasonable basis for assuming that he gives promise of the successful completion of the training and preparation, of attaining the desired training, qualification, or skill, and of becoming a "necessary man" in an activity necessary to war production or essential to the support of the war effort.[20]

Over the course of the war, the criteria for drafting men changed. Experience showed that the younger the recruit, the better the individual could meet military requirements. In November 1942, Congress passed an amendment to the Selective Training and Service Act dropping the age of draft eligibility to eighteen.

In November 1942, Bernard V. Christensen wrote to H. C. Newton, then president of AACP and dean of the Massachusetts College of Pharmacy, in response to a request for information on the status of students. Speaking for Ohio State, Christensen reported that four students had enlisted since the end of September 1942, that 133 men remained enrolled and that, of these, fifty-one were currently deferred, including twenty-four who had enlisted in the Reserves. Christensen noted that the local draft boards had been reasonable about deferments for juniors and seniors.

I think this is due somewhat to the fact that the Office of the State Director of Selective Service issued a special bulletin to local boards with reference to Federal Selective Service Memorandum, I-62. Last summer we had some difficulty due to the fact that local boards had the impression that I-62 had been canceled. Upon calling this to the attention of the State Director, he contacted the federal office and found out that I-62 was still in force. Consequently, he advised local boards accordingly, and since that time their attitude has been less critical.[21]

The War Manpower Commission was a policymaking agency established in April 1942. Although the War Manpower Commission tried to establish policy on draft deferments, Selective Service functioned as a separate agency. The Committee on War Activities of the American Pharmaceutical Association, made up of C. R. Bohrer, A. G. DuMez, and Robert Fischelis, served as the pharmacy liaison with the Division of Professional and Technical Personnel of the War Manpower Commission. The committee wrote to Dr. Edward C. Elliott requesting deferment for pharmacy students such that 1,750 students would still graduate each year. This level was based on the average graduation rate of the prewar years and the decline in student populations. Elliott, the president of Purdue University and also the chief of the division, requested pharmacy demographic information.* The Army estimated the need for 5,100 pharmacists for an Army of 3,600,000, the objective for 1942. Similarly, the Navy estimated a need of 2,800 pharmacists for its force of 750,000 men. The total forces were estimated to reach 9 million men by the end of 1943. The committee used the 1940 U.S. Census data to argue that providing the military with the 15,000 pharmacists to meet the estimated needs of the expanded Army and Navy by the end of 1943 would be impossible without grave consequences to the civilian population. The authors pressed for the institution of a selection process that could identify those pharmacists needed in the community and those who could be drafted without risking loss of pharmaceutical services to the civilian population. They recommended that each state's Selective Ser-

---

*In 1947, Edward C. Elliott, the president emeritus of Purdue University, was selected to lead the landmark pharmaceutical survey which would become known as the Elliott Report. The survey was sponsored by the American Council on Education.

vice office work with a state-level pharmacy advisory committee to determine who the necessary men were. Some states had already implemented such an advisory body. Maryland's advisory committee, formed on February 15, 1942, had already reviewed 126 applicants, recommending less than 25 percent for deferment as necessary men.[22]

The Committee on War Activities held a series of meetings with Elliott and the Selective Service in an attempt to obtain a deferment for pharmacy students. On February 13, 1943, Elliott informed the committee that "no plans had been made nor were any contemplated in the future by the War Manpower Commission for the deferment of any pharmacy students."[23] In what appeared to be the final option, the committee approached Secretary of War Henry L. Stimson with the statement that the "life of approximately 65 colleges of pharmacy and consequently an adequate supply of pharmacists for military and civilian requirements is at stake."[24] The committee requested that pharmacy education be integrated with military instruction, as medicine and dentistry were. The secretary of war refused, stating that "the Army was able to secure all the pharmacists that it required through the operation of the draft and that an Army program for the education of pharmacists was, therefore, not needed."[25] Charles H. Rogers, chair of the Executive Committee of AACP, also addressed a lengthy letter to Elliott, again setting out the dire consequences to the colleges and the public if a sufficient number of students did not receive deferment until they had completed their full course of education.

On May 1, 1943, national pharmacy organizations (AACP, ACPE, APhA, NABP, and NARD) developed a brief for the War Manpower Commission titled "In Support of the Continued Classification of Pharmacy As an Essential Activity Under Health and Welfare Service, the Continued Deferment of Pharmacists, and a Provision for the Training of an Adequate Number of Pharmacists." The brief stated that the current level of deferment for pharmacists had been reasonably satisfactory and that this level needed to be maintained as the available civilian pool of registered pharmacists continued to shrink. The crux of the problem, however, was student deferments and the declining supply of new graduates. A review of the enrollment data revealed that the schools would be able to supply less than 40 percent of the anticipated replacement needs. In spite of deferments for some students and the acceleration of the curriculum to three years, there was a decrease of more than 55 percent in enrollments in the 1942-1943 academic year. Over 1,500 students left school in 1942-1943 for military service.[26]

Selective Service issued Occupational Bulletin #11 on March 1, 1943. This provided deferment until July 1, 1943, for those pharmacy students who were juniors or seniors, that is, halfway through their professional education. All other students were immediately subject to the draft. Students in chemistry and physics were deferred until July of 1945 on the condition that they could finish their degrees within that time frame. Students who were in premedical, predental, or preveterinary programs and qualified for admission to a professional school were also draft exempt until July 1945.[27] Within several months the bulletin was revised and reissued as Occupational Bulletin #33-6; the revision included pharmacy students. To qualify for deferment, the college had to document that the student was competent to complete the course and would graduate within twenty-four months. In addition, the number of freshmen the college could admit was limited to 150 percent of the graduating classes for the years 1940 to 1943.

Colleges of pharmacy worked to have students deferred, at least until they could graduate. For many schools, retaining students was a matter of survival as enrollments continued to shrink. The Selective Service Activity and Occupational Bulletin #33-6 addressed deferments for students in pharmacy, forestry, optometry, and agricultural sciences. However, the bulletin was only an advisory to the local boards. The APhA War Emergency Advisory Committee was particularly active in trying to gain a blanket deferment for pharmacy students.

Although the pharmacy press and the professional organizations continued to support the deferment of students, their efforts were hampered because of the perception of pharmacy by the military and by the officials in the War Manpower Commission and Selective Service. The latter two were interested in understanding the consequences of a diminished supply of pharmacists, as evidenced by the series of meetings with pharmacy committees. Elliott explained the War Manpower Commission's reluctance to expand pharmacy student deferment based on the lack of awareness of the pharmacist's role as a health care professional, the concentration of drugstores in cities (giving the appearance of excess supply), and the lack of proof of a national shortage of pharmacists. He also added that a difference of opinion existed in Washington as to the probable length of the war and the need to maintain training of professionals for future needs.[28]

In the 1943 report of the APhA War Emergency Advisory Committee, Chairman Andrew DuMez gave a blunt assessment of the difficulty in obtaining deferments for pharmacy students on the same basis as physicians:

1. The ratio of pharmacists in the armed forces to the total number of practicing pharmacists is far below that of either physicians or dentists;
2. there are no authentic statistics to show there is an overall shortage of pharmacists or that the pharmaceutical service now available to the public is inadequate; and,
3. the non-professional appearance of the average drugstore and the commercial nature of its predominant activities.[29]

Robert Fischelis, in a long personal letter dated July 3, 1943, told Rufus Lyman of his work with the Office of Civilian Requirements in the War Production Board, which was responsible for the oversight of essential civilian supplies and service. He informed Lyman that he had received a request from the War Manpower Commission for information on the pharmacy situation and the deferment of pharmacy students. He shared the perception of individuals in Selective Service and the War Manpower Commission that pharmacy had failed to make its case. There were too many pharmacies in areas of high visibility to decision makers and the "slapstick atmosphere of the front of their drugstores" did not impress observers with the professional function of the pharmacists. In a candid moment, he shared his belief that a twenty-four-month deferment was the best that anyone could hope for or request. He acknowledged that the superacceleration program was a difficult choice but the best one given war conditions and requirements.[30]

Many of the colleges were troubled by decreased enrollments. Freshmen entry classes decreased in numbers as young men entered the military right out of high school or went to work in war production plants. The situation was equally bleak as upperclassmen left either because of the draft or enlistment. By the fall of 1943 total enrollment had fallen to 3,546 with 940 potential graduates.[31]

In the total educational environment, students and educational institutions were treated relatively gently by the draft system. Until the buildup for the invasion of France, many draft boards were generous with student deferrals. This changed by mid-1944; less than 10,000 college deferments were granted nationally.[32]

NECESSARY MEN

The Selective Training and Service Act of 1940 first established the deferment mechanism for "those men whose employment in industry, agriculture, or other occupations or employment, or whose activity in other endeavors is found . . . to be necessary to the maintenance of the National health, safety or interest."[33] Individuals determined to be necessary men were to be classified II-A. The regulations governing this part of the legislation defines the necessary man and the general criteria for granting such a designation:

> A registrant shall be considered a "necessary man" in industry, business, employment, agricultural pursuit, governmental service, or in any other service or endeavor, including training and preparation therefore, only when all of these conditions exist:
> a. He is, or but for a seasonal or temporary interruption would be engaged in such an activity.
> b. He cannot be replaced satisfactorily because of a shortage of persons with his qualifications or skill in such activity.
> c. His removal would cause a material loss of effectiveness in such activity.[34]

There are no Selective Service records of the number of necessary men who were exempted from the draft. The decision for such status was usually at the discretion of the local draft board, and these records were not collected or maintained at the conclusion of the war.

The Selective Service Activity and Occupation Bulletin #32 addressed the subject of civilian health and welfare services with a focus on physicians, dentists, and veterinarians. Part II identified essential activities, and "pharmaceutical services" were listed among these activities. Part III of the bulletin enumerated essential occupations. Pharmacy was listed and defined:

> This title includes only those persons who are licensed to practice pharmacy in conformance with State laws; who are actively engaged in the practice of pharmacy, and whose professional services are available on a full-time basis. It does not include pharmacists when engaged in other than the practice of pharmacy, or other persons who may be employed in a pharmacy or drugstore.[35]

The Oregon State Board was reported as using this bulletin as a central part of a pamphlet mailed to all draft boards in the state. The pamphlet stated that 36 percent of the state's physicians were already in uniform, a fact which required pharmacists to assume new responsibilities as health care providers. While the pamphlet was ostensibly to provide information for an informed decision on draftee selection, the conclusion took an adversarial stance by putting the draft boards on notice. "Obviously, we wish to absolve ourselves of contemplated charges of gross negligence in the event the drugstores of the state are unable to render adequate pharmaceutical services should an epidemic or other emergency endanger public health."[36]

In general, the process of declaring a man necessary was that, upon the receipt of his draft notice (and not before), the employer was required to request deferment on the basis of the individual being necessary to the enterprise. The employer's request was required to include

- a full job description,
- a statement of the shortage of skills that the man was employed for,
- the fact that the employee's removal would cause material loss of productivity, and
- the required time to train or recruit a replacement.

In addition, the employer was required to provide a statement of his goods and services and why they were essential to the well-being of the community or the nation. This question helped determine whether the business itself was essential to the war effort because, by extension, if the business was not necessary the man could not be either.

Thus, the individual was not in a position to request consideration as a necessary man—his employer had to do it. Employers were prohibited from requesting deferment unless the individual agreed to it. David Powers, a 1939 graduate of Columbia, recalled being called a draft dodger as he commuted between Brooklyn and Manhattan. He discovered that his employer had submitted requests to have him declared a necessary man without his knowledge. When Powers discovered this, he volunteered for the draft and ended up in the Air Corps as a navigator in B24s. He completed twenty-five combat missions in the European Theater of Operations and retired as a major.[37]

Whether an individual was a necessary man or not was frequently difficult for a local draft board to determine, especially in the case of pharmacy. Were all pharmacists automatically necessary? If not, which were and which were not?

PHARMACY ADVISORY COMMITTEES

The establishment of state pharmacy advisory committees to help identify those men who were necessary to the health of their communities was a major agenda item when thirty-two state secretaries and other state association officials met with APhA staff and government officials in Washington, DC, on February 20 and 21, 1942. In 1943, the National Headquarters of Selective Service notified the state offices that they could confer with special committees to help in that decision process.[38] The committees were advisory only; their function was to gather information and provide it to Selective Service so that a qualified decision could be made. The advisory committees considered information such as the amount of prescription service provided within a community and, if a store had to be closed because a pharmacist was drafted, whether other stores could assume the professional volume.[39]

The advisory committee was usually organized to include representatives from the state pharmacy association, board, and college(s). In addition, a representative of the state Selective Service office was assigned to the committee. The committee communicated directly with the state Selective Service office; it had no official contact with local draft boards.[40]

Numerous references to pharmacy advisory committees in the pharmacy press of the day stated that committees were being established or were authorized. These advisory committees were not an official part of any larger governmental or professional organization. Their deliberations were sensitive since their recommendations had the potential to send a man from his community into combat and even death. However, there is every indication that the committees were active and provided a useful service.

In 1943 APhA staff asked the state association secretaries to list the individuals serving on the advisory committee in their states. At least thirty-nine states responded with individual names and addresses of committee members; several cautioned that the information was confidential and not to be released under any condition (see Appendix II). In the Connecticut response dated August 9, 1943, Hugh P. Bierne added a note stating, "This committee has been functioning for 15 months. Have had upwards of 200 appeals referred. In this time the State Selective headquarters have rejected our recommendations but twice."[41]

The pharmacy organizations in each state developed their own procedures for establishing an advisory committee and working with the state Selective Service. Some of the states had a relatively small committee with the identities of the individuals kept confidential. Other states attempted to have committee members represent specific locations in the state. Almost all states had representatives from the college of pharmacy, the state board, and the state association on the committee. The level of interaction between the various advisory committees and the state Selective Service office also varied. Several states were particularly proactive in their work.

The New York Advisory Committee

New York's committee undertook a two-part process to determine the number of active pharmacists and the portion of their time spent providing essential pharmaceutical services. Approximately 5,500 pharmacists responded to the survey. With the help of the A. C. Nielsen Company, senior pharmacy students from the six New York colleges of pharmacy visited 100 sample drugstores and spent one to two days tabulating the minute-by-minute activities of pharmacists. The New York Selective Service office issued Occupational Memorandum #23 noting that occupational deferment should be given to pharmacists when their removal from the community would impair the public interest.[42]

The Illinois Advisory Committee

In Illinois the advisory committee surveyed the state to ascertain the number and distribution of active pharmacists to aid in identifying which pharmacists were necessary men. Based on the results, the advisory committee determined that the ratio of one pharmacist to 1,500 people in cities and one to 1,800 in rural areas was the level necessary to provide adequate services. In order to identify essential drugstores, the committee developed a test based on public health sales. The sales of the fountain, tobacco, toiletries, magazines and newspapers, cameras, and sundries were subtracted from the total sales; the rest of the store's sales were considered to be public health items. The amount of public health sales was used to set a standard for how many pharmacists might be considered necessary; sales of less than $15,000 per year would justify only one pharmacist; sales over $15,000 might justify more than one. The Illinois Advisory Committee reported that as of July 1943, 25 percent of the requests for recommendation for deferment were turned down. The state Selective Service office approved of this system and notified local Illinois draft boards in Memorandum #568 that information was available to help them determine the proper classification of pharmacists.[43] A postwar history of the Illinois Selective Service acknowledged the contributions of the advisory committee in helping local boards fairly and properly determine the draft classification of pharmacists.[44]

The New Jersey Pharmacy Advisory Committee

The New Jersey Pharmacy Advisory Committee's administrative officer was Robert Fischelis, who also represented the Board of Pharmacy. Ernest Little, dean of the College of Pharmacy; John Debus, secretary of the state association; and five other pharmacists constituted the committee, along with Major, later Colonel, Schwehm, a nonpharmacist representative of the New Jersey Selective Service office.* It was agreed that, while the committee's role was to provide assistance to local boards, all requests for deferral as "necessary men" must be funneled through the state Selective Service office. Schwehm defined "necessary" to include the activity as well as the man in preserving public health. Once a man had been deferred, he could not change his job and keep the deferment. The procedure would have to be repeated to determine whether the new practice site was essential and whether he was a necessary man in it. The basis for determining an individual's necessity was discussed, and the principles were agreed upon. They include the following:

> Number of pharmacists available for service in a pharmacy
> Number of pharmacists in a particular area
> Number of pharmacists available for military service in that area
> Number of pharmacies available for public service[45]

The committee did not consider many students in the course of its fourteen meetings. As mentioned, Selective Service was precluded from deferring a complete category, such as students or pharmacists. During the second meeting, held on July 30, 1943, several students were discussed and deferment recommended. Deferment for a limited period was also recommended to allow those who were eligible to take the board the time to do so. However, there was no deferment to allow pharmacy interns to complete the time required for them to be eligible to take the state board examination. During this same meeting, criteria were established to determine whether a relief man could be considered a necessary man. The criteria were that

- the relief clerk must work five days a week, fifty hours per week;
- the weekly schedule, including stores covered, must be filed with the board of pharmacy; and
- information must be verified with employer's records.

---

* The New Jersey Pharmacy Advisory Committee for Selective Service was established on June 11, 1943, and disbanded on May 26, 1944. The minutes for all fourteen meetings of the committee, with the exception of August 13, 1943, are in the Fischelis files. The minutes contain information about committee organization, procedural items, and the names of 205 men who were considered for recommendation as necessary men to the Selective Service. With few exceptions, there is little information to indicate why deferment was or was not recommended. Robert P. Fischelis Papers, AACP files, American Institute of the History of Pharmacy Collection housed at the Wisconsin Historical Society, Madison,Wisconsin, Mss 619, Box 188, f2.

The New Jersey records do offer specific illustrations that provide some insights into the process. For example, Jacob H. Cohen was a relief pharmacist who covered two drugstores. He was considered and recommended for deferment as a necessary man. He was periodically reviewed during almost every meeting of the committee, his status reconfirmed, and his recommendation for deferment upheld.

In another instance, that of Phillip J. Maffey, registered pharmacist, the recommendation said "the report of the investigation of a representative of the committee was given consideration, and it was unanimously agreed that he not be recommended for deferment as a necessary man." The wording is almost identical in the case of Richard Henches, registered pharmacist-owner, except it ends "that he be recommended for deferment as a necessary man."[46]

Frequently, no reason was given when the decision was not to recommend deferment. However, in at least two cases there is documentation that the recommendation was based on the practice site not being essential to the health of the community.

Sidney Silverman was an employee pharmacist for a drugstore owner who was too ill to work. A registered pharmacist was required to keep the store licensed as a drugstore. The recommendation was that Silverman not be deferred based on the fact that while the employee pharmacist was essential to the continuing operation of the store, the store itself was not essential to the health and welfare of the community.[47,48]

Vincent L. Mascia, an employed pharmacist of the Liggett Drug Co., was not recommended for deferment.[49] In January 1944, the state Selective Service requested review of his status when the pharmacist moved to a different Liggett drugstore. Selective Service voiced concern that such transfers might result in "unfair deferment procedures."[50] The committee again did not recommend deferment. Finally, by the tenth meeting, Vincent L. Mascia had become employed at the Davis Pharmacy in Hackensack. With this change in practice site, he was recommended for deferment as a necessary man.[51]

Being an owner did not mean an automatic deferment. The situation for William Einhorn, registered pharmacist-owner, is recorded in the last meeting of 1943 and the first of 1944. Lee Drug filled 5,400 prescriptions in 1942, and 70 percent of the store's business was in medicines and drugs.[52] Einhorn had an employee pharmacist of approximately the same age and draft status. Further examination showed that while the store was in the vicinity of several war industries, employees from the plants did not use the pharmacy in the evenings and thus it was believed that one pharmacist could handle the prescription volume. Since Mr. Einhorn had received a draft call and the other pharmacist had not, the decision of the committee was that it would be unfair to defer Einhorn at the potential expense of the employee pharmacist. The committee voted not to recommend deferment of Einhorn as a necessary man.[53]

The fourteenth meeting of the advisory committee was held on May 26, 1944. The Selective Service notified the committee that draft quotas were set and it was unlikely that additional meetings would be needed. The New Jersey Pharmacy Advisory Committee had reviewed the cases of 205 men during the year that it met. Of these, 102 men were recommended for deferment, and ninety-three were not. The others received no action or a recommendation for limited deferment. At least six men who were not recommended for deferment eventually entered the service (Gerald Burstein, Nicholas Dmytriw, Samuel Kitikoff, Anthony S. Ordille, Joseph M. Puhan, and Jerry A. Rosa). In addition, at least one man who was recommended for deferment ended up in the military (Irving Bloomfield).

The bulk of the committee's deliberations were about pharmacists who were practicing retail pharmacy in New Jersey. However, other considerations were undertaken at the request of Selective Service, including an individual who practiced in New Jersey but whose residence and draft board were in New York.[54] Selective Service also requested the committee's help to review several nonpharmacists who were involved in pharmacy.

The experience of Richard Farrow, a 1937 graduate of the Philadelphia College of Pharmacy, illustrates how the process worked and the consequences, which could be tragic. Farrow entered the Army on May 11, 1942. After training he served for a short stint as a pharmacist and was then transferred to Officers Candidate School in the Medical Administrative Corps. He "washed out" and returned to Fort Meade.[55] In 1944 Richard Farrow applied for honorable discharge as a necessary man. His father, a pharmacist owner, had died, and Farrow wanted to take over his store. Richard's wife was running the store with the help of a registered pharmacist. The local board asked Selective Service to review this application, and the question was referred to the advisory committee.[56] The case was considered on the same basis as if the individual was not yet in the service. The conclusion was that if the requestor was currently managing his father's pharmacy he would not be recommended as a necessary man because the store was not necessary to the health and welfare of the community.[57] Richard Farrow was assigned to a medical detachment of an infantry division and shipped overseas in November 1944. He was killed in action in Germany on February 7, 1945.[58]

ACCOMMODATIONS

The colleges had a high level of interest in doing something for the students who went into the service before they finished their college education; this attitude extended to those who had not fulfilled the requirement for practical experience. Ohio State University, for example, allowed those who were called into the military or other war-essential activities after the midpoint of the term to receive full credit for all courses in which they had a satisfactory record. In the case of seniors, full credit would be allowed if they were called up during the month before graduation. In all cases the final grade would be awarded at the discretion of the professor. Ohio State also announced that any student who returned after the war could receive up to fifteen credit hours for military experience and, if the student was within fifteen credit hours of graduation, could graduate. However, in the case of professional curricula, such as pharmacy, these credits could be granted only if they did not conflict with the appropriate licensing body.[59] The state board's attitude toward this accommodation was tested when a student lacking nine hours toward graduation petitioned for the credits to be waived. The response from the board was that all requirements had to be met before a degree would be granted, and that a school granting a degree when the course work was not completed "subjects the college to being stricken from the list of recognized colleges of pharmacy."[60]

Some states held special board examinations for those who were going into the military and therefore unable to take them at the usual time.[61] Marvin Segel is an example of how state boards accommodated the young men departing for military service. Segel was called to active duty on June 15, 1942, his graduation day from Ohio State. He was able to take his board exam on June 16 and 17 but had to be in uniform since he was on active duty. He remembered that

> every member of the board came over, looked over my shoulder, pointed to the questions that I had wrongly answered and asked me to reread the question (even the true and false ones). At the end of the exam the President of the Board put his arm around me and said "don't worry son, when you get out of the service, you will have a license."[62]

Among the boards a core issue was the problem men would face gaining reciprocity at a later date. If a man gained a license under special conditions, that license might not be acceptable to another state. For example, some states required that the individual attain age twenty-one before taking the board examinations, while others stipulated only that the license could not be issued until age twenty-one. Some states did not allow candidates to take the examination until all of the requirements for licensure were complete. In Missouri this included one year of experience and being twenty-one years old. Other states, including Florida, allowed individuals to take the boards but held the license until the man reached the necessary age or completed the experience requirement, either in the military or upon his return from the service. Illinois allowed the individual to take the written part of the examination immediately after graduation and the practical after the requisite internship was completed.[63] This age requirement became more critical as a consequence of the accelerated three-year academic programs. NABP members were reminded of the resolution to grant reciprocity whenever it was legal and to be as liberal as possible in determining a candidate's request.[64]

Patrick Costello, secretary of the National Association of Boards of Pharmacy, raised the issue of reciprocal exchange of licenses between states and urged care on the part of both colleges and states when considering changes that might endanger the interstate agreements. He pointed out that one state could change the requirements for age or practical experience; however, if other states did not make similar accommodations it would be impossible for pharmacists to reciprocate their licenses later. He suggested that graduating seniors should be careful to meet the maximum requirements for licensure rather than the minimum. He noted that several states had already voided the age requirement but explained that individuals taking advantage of that exemption would be unable to reciprocate to states that maintained the age requirement—even if the second state passed a similar exemption later.[65] For example, Jefferson Franklyn Pickard of Greensboro, North Carolina, graduated before he was twenty-one years old but was allowed to take his board examinations before he left for the Navy. In the letter notifying him that he had passed, F. W. Hancock, the secretary-treasurer of the board, added a handwritten note that the license would not be issued until Pickard reached age twenty-one—and the license would be so dated.[66]

In Michigan the attorney general suggested that it would be appropriate during the war emergency to suspend the requirement that only graduates be allowed to sit for the state exam. Instead, he suggested, anyone who was reasonably sure to graduate within sixty days should be allowed to take the exam.[67] The problem this type of exception could cause for reciprocity was later apparent when Stuart Price of Michigan was refused reciprocity to Ohio. Price had completed all of the graduation requirements and taken his boards before formal graduation, a practice not allowed in that state.[68]

Chapter 4

The Drugstore in the War Effort

> The drugstore is an American institution, a democratic institution known to no other part of the world.[1]

In his APhA presidential address in August 1941, Charles Evans' sentiment about the centrality of the drugstore in American life left no ambiguity. He noted that the pharmacist was looked upon as a community leader, the one person to whom young and old go for information and advice, and he added that their stores were the meeting places of all people. Thus the professional leadership set the expectation that pharmacy understood it had an obligation to the general welfare of the community and the country.

December 7, 1941, brought an immediate change to life in the United States. The retail business of pharmacy was affected as were all other retail businesses. The attack on Pearl Harbor brought the war closer than it had seemed before, especially to those on the coasts. Enemy submarines were reported close to both the Atlantic and Pacific coasts; blackout regulations were established in anticipation of an enemy air raid. In Connecticut, NARD President Hugh Bierne pledged to the governor the assistance of every druggist and drugstore in the state. Every Connecticut druggist had been supplied with a list of poisons and instructions of what to do and whom to contact if any stranger attempted to purchase them. This precaution addressed a concern over the safety of public water supplies.

George Frates, chairman of the NARD executive committee, reported on a San Francisco blackout in response to the report of enemy aircraft on December 12. All lights were turned off and no cars moved in San Francisco from 7:30 to 10:00 p.m. when the all clear was sounded. On the evening of December 18 over 1,200 druggists and salespeople attended a Red Cross meeting, the largest gathering of San Francisco druggists ever. Over 300 druggists signed up to take first-aid courses. Owners pledged to outfit a first-aid kit at their own expense and furnish it to an emergency center whenever it was needed.[2]

In April 1942 *Drug Topics* presented a snapshot (see Table 4.1) of the involvement of the nation's drugstores in the war effort to that date.[3]

CIVIL DEFENSE

Many pharmacists who wanted to be involved quickly volunteered to make their stores an emergency aid station. The drugstore offered many advantages, including a ready supply of first-aid products and pharmacists. However, the Office of Civilian Defense (OCD) discouraged the use of a drugstore as an aid station, largely based on experience gained during bombings in Britain. Some saw the position of the Office of Civilian Defense as a rebuff; they felt pharmacists should be free to establish first-aid centers if they wished.

TABLE 4.1. Drugstore War Contributions Through March 1942

The Record	Independents	Chains	Totals
Number of stores	54,912	5,276	60,188
Number of stores selling defense stamps	40,681	5,181	45,862
Total value of defense stamps sold	$14,135,622	$8,590,098	$22,725,720
Number of owners and clerks in United States (full-time and part-time)	191,642	64,894	256,536
Number of owners/clerks with first-aid certificates	33,192	2,382	35,574
Number of owners/clerks taking first-aid courses	59,936	6,231	66,167
Number of owners/clerks in the armed forces	13,473	5,170	18,643
Pounds of collapsible tin collected	299,817	32,321	332,138

John W. McPherrin, editor in chief of *American Druggist* and outspoken advocate for pharmacy, used his influence at the magazine to set the record straight on the issue of civilian defense. He provided space to George Baehr, the chief medical officer of OCD, to explain the OCD's cool reception to using pharmacies as first-aid centers. Baehr complimented the desire of pharmacists to help but noted that the blitz in Britain made shambles of drugstores with their large expanse of windows and shelves full of glass packaging. He observed that the restricted amount of floor space in the modern drugstore did not allow for treatment of large numbers of victims and explained the need to concentrate victims into a triage system where the necessary records of injuries and treatment could be facilitated.[4] He noted that the OCD must be prepared to provide first aid in response to an enemy attack that involves many, not a peace-time first aid effort involving one or two individuals. In an accompanying story, *American Druggist* reported that the OCD plan was well founded on facts, not bureaucracy, and encouraged pharmacists to become involved.[5]

The Office of Civilian Defense, with the assistance of pharmacists, prepared a manual for pharmacists involved in first aid and other civilian defense activities. The manual stated that casualties needed to receive care in a casualty station or first-aid post but acknowledged that many Americans thought of the drugstore first in an emergency and would go there to seek aid. A sixteen-point plan was provided; the first suggestion was for pharmacists to gain certification in a Red Cross first-aid class. Other suggestions included becoming an information center for OCD materials and assisting in authorized first-aid posts. A list of contents for an emergency supply kit was provided; pharmacists were encouraged to discuss the contents with the local chief of emergency services. Items ranged from bandaging supplies and materials to medications, especially for burns and wound cleansing. In addition, pharmacies were encouraged to keep on hand adequate stocks of emergency medicines for physicians' use. Items suggested included tetanus antitoxin, ethyl chloride, ampuls of caffeine sodio-benzoate, hypodermic tablets of morphine sulfate, ether for anesthesia, aromatic spirits of ammonia (pearls), and tannic acid.[6] Pharmacy associations developed a qualification program. The stores that met the requirements were given a placard bearing the official civil defense logo which indicated registration as a pharmaceutical unit.

Pharmacists quickly began to participate in the program. The Ohio Valley Druggist Association raised funds to purchase the recommended supplies and medicines for each of the area's twenty-eight casualty stations. (The anticipated cost of these materials in 1942 was forty-three dollars.) The requirements for listing as a pharmaceutical unit included providing information on the number of pharmacists employed in the store and identifying those qualified in first aid; procuring the supplies and medicines identified in the civilian defense manual; and promising to comply with the requirements of OCD.[7]

Massachusetts pharmacies, with the approval of OCD, established auxiliary emergency medical depots in many stores. This program included a locked cabinet of the materials identified in the civilian defense manual with access restricted to air-raid wardens, doctors, and nurses. Stores had to be certified by the state board before receiving the designation as a depot.[8]

CIVILIAN HEALTH

Labor, or manpower, was as much an issue on the civilian scene as it was in the military. Workers were urgently needed in the war production industries to turn out the arms and materials required by the rapidly increasing American military and its allies. In 1942 alone 3.75 million workers were moved from civilian to military production; the number of unemployed shrank from 3.8 million to 1.5 million. By the end of 1942 the average workweek in manufacturing was over forty-four hours; in the shipbuilding and aircraft industries it was over forty-seven hours.[9] In his book *Why the Allies Won* Richard Overy described American mass production as an important advantage. He noted that American industry manufactured almost two-thirds of the total allied military equipment that was produced during the war. By 1943 Kaiser shipyards had reduced the time to build Liberty ships from 1.4 million work hours and 355 days to less than 500,000 work hours and 41 days. The last civilian automobile came off the line on February 10, 1942; only 139 automobiles were built in Detroit for the remainder of the war. By 1944 Ford was producing one B-24 bomber every sixty-three minutes at its Willow Run facility.[10]

Recognizing that the health of the production workers was as critical as the health of the armed forces, the government established a branch of the War Production Board to oversee civilians' health needs. Pharmacist Fred J. Stock was named to head the effort. This branch was responsible for the production, allocation, and supply of all medicines for both military and civilians throughout World War II.

The civilian challenge was keeping worker sickness and accidents to a minimum, thus avoiding lost production time. One estimate reported in the pharmacy literature was that 1 million workers were absent every working day because of illnesses and accidents, many of which could have been prevented. The chief culprits were colds and other respiratory problems, poor diet, unspecified contagious diseases, toothaches and other dental problems, and infections due to untended cuts and scrapes. Pharmacists participated in the prevention and treatment of these ailments by promoting and selling first aid and proprietary products. Pharmacists were exhorted to work with physicians, dentists, and nurses to keep Americans healthy and on the job.[11]

BOND DRIVES

World War II was expensive for the United States treasury; postwar estimates were that the total cost exceeded $350 billion. The U.S. Treasury was charged with procuring the necessary funds. Both personal and corporate income taxes were increased. Funds were also raised from other taxing sources including production, use, and sales taxes. The second part of the treasury's challenge was to keep inflation under control. More people were working and wages were increasing; the economic constraints of the Great Depression were over. However, fewer goods and services were available to satisfy consumer demand. The combination of excess cash and fewer goods was recognized as a formula for price increases and inflation.[12]

One solution to the problem of surplus cash was to convince the public to purchase war bonds. Besides being an answer to the treasury's cash challenge, the purchase of war bonds also gave men and women on the home front a more personal role in the war effort. Eight general war bond (also called war loan) drives were held between late 1942 and the end of 1945. The bond drives were designed to appeal to individual citizens rather than banks or other financial organizations.

The drives often had multiple collection points, including employers, municipalities, and retail establishments. Pharmacies were an important part of the various bond drives.

The nation's drugstores sold Defense Stamps even before the United States declared war. *Drug Topics* reported that almost $23 million of war savings stamps were sold in 45,862 pharmacies between May 1, 1941, and March 1, 1942. This was 16.5 percent of all stamps sold through all channels for the period.[13] Based on the success of that drive, the treasury devised a new program, concentrating stamp sales in a single industry: pharmacy—called the "drug trade"—was selected as the first sponsor in the belief that a successful campaign would lead to similar programs in other fields.

The drug trade included every facet of pharmacy. Independent and chain drugstores were represented, as were drug and cosmetic manufacturers, wholesalers, and advertising agencies. John W. McPherrin, editor in chief of *American Druggist,* was named as the general chairman representing the treasury; his vice chair was Jennings Murphy, secretary of the Wisconsin State Pharmaceutical Association and chair of the National Conference of Pharmaceutical Secretaries. Each group was given a specific role to play in the campaign. The advertising community was charged with preparing promotional materials for manufacturers to include in their normal promotions to drugstores. A general theme of "Bullets 25¢ a Dozen at Your Drugstore" was developed. The logo for the drive depicted a colonial minuteman with a musket in his right hand and his left resting on his plow. Advertising included radio spots, newspapers, and popular magazines. Point-of-sale materials were developed for use in drugstores. Manufacturers' sales representatives helped retailers prepare window and store displays and promoted the participation of all their customers. Wholesalers distributed the stamps to their retail customers, saving the retailer the trip to the post office to purchase them.

The campaign was scheduled to run during May. The pharmacy press, both national and regional, ran stories about the need for drugstores to make the campaign a success. The *Apothecary,* a regional magazine in the Northeast, editorialized that the entire population, all 130 million, was some druggist's customer and that selling them war stamps was a form of everyday civilian defense service.[14] The *Southeastern Drug Journal* noted that the success of the drive, based on the presence of drugstores in every community, would set an example for future drives.[15] The *NARD Journal* printed a nine-point marketing plan in support of the promotion, urging owners to make the program the most heavily advertised product in the store. The journal also noted that this national promotion would direct customers to the drugstore, and that no other retailer, not even grocery stores, would enjoy the advantages of this promotion.[16] *American Druggist* reprinted an editorial that appeared in many of the Hearst newspapers under the title "Behind the Men Behind the Guns." The editorial explained that the program was designed to make it as easy for the American public to buy a war savings stamp as it was to buy a toothbrush. It concluded that "if ALL our lines of related industry and trade will do as the druggists are doing, there need be no more talk of 'compulsory' war savings in a free America."[17]

The results of the stamp drive, announced in July 1942, were impressive. Sales totaled over 7.25 million dollars, more than 4 percent of all retail drugstore sales in May. Over 70 percent of independent and 90 percent of chain stores participated in the drive. The advertising campaign's cost was estimated to exceed $200,000; however, most of the services and materials were donated. In the final accounting, the total out-of-pocket expense was $16,000. The national pharmacy associations contributed the funds to cover all costs.[18]

Pharmacists were involved in a number of local bond campaigns. Some sold bonds for military equipment, such as bombers.[19] The Queens County Pharmacists of New York announced a "Build-A-Sub" bond campaign with a goal of $7 million.[20] Over 700 retail pharmacists participated in the drive which lasted only one month and exceeded the goal by over $500,000.[21,22] The submarine, the USS *Besugo* (SS-321), was commissioned on June 19, 1944.*

In 1943 Fred Felter, editor of the regional *Pacific Drug Review,* suggested that pharmacists again participate collectively in a bond drive. He suggested that funds be collected to purchase C-47 Douglas ambulance planes. Other regional and state pharmacy journals joined

---

*The *Besugo* received four battle stars for World War II service. She made five war patrols in the Bungo and Makassar Straits, South China and Java Seas. On April 23, 1945, she sank the German submarine, U-183. *Bungo* also served during the Korean War and received an additional battle star. The *Bungo* was sold for scrap in 1976. Mooney, J. L. (Ed.) (1959). *Dictionary of American Naval Fighting Ships.* Washington, DC: Naval Historical Center, Department of the Navy, GPO, p. 121.

in espousing the campaign. Connecticut pharmacists tested the plan later in 1943. Finally, after sustained prodding from the regional journals, NARD agreed to support the project editorially in its journal.[23,24]

The ambulance plane drive was scheduled to be part of the 4th War Loan Drive, running January 18 to February 29, 1944. It was required that the state pharmacy association be the sponsor; national or regional organizations were not eligible. All drugstores sales of "E" series bonds would be credited to the drive. Pharmacists, customers,

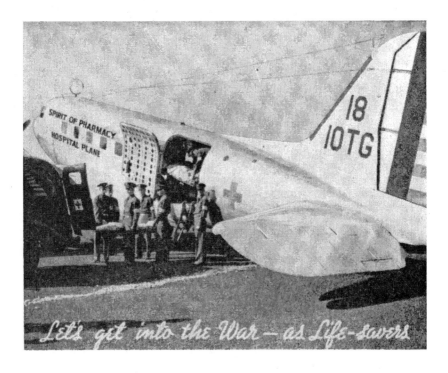

In 1943 Fred Felter, editor of the regional journal *Pacific Drug Review,* suggested that pharmacists sell bonds to purchase C-47 Douglas ambulance planes. Other regional and state pharmacy journals joined in espousing the campaign. Connecticut pharmacists tested the plan later in 1943. More than fifty-four planes were purchased through the drive that ran from January 18 to February 29, 1944. (*Source: The Apothecary* [1942] 54:32. Photo courtesy of the Lloyd Library and Museum.)

wholesalers, or manufacturers could buy bonds, but in order to count toward the purchase of the ambulance plane the purchase had to be through a drugstore. The goal of the drive was to purchase a Douglas C-47, the military version of the DC-3, that was equipped to carry medical supplies and personnel into combat zones and ferry the wounded out. They would also be used to ferry wounded soldiers in the continental United States. Each plane cost $147,500 of "E" bond face value; state pharmacy associations that raised the total sum could name the plane for their organization. If funds were raised for additional planes, other district or city pharmacy organizations would have naming rights.[25]

In spite of concerns over the sum that needed to be raised, the campaign was a success. Arkansas druggists sold over $1.2 million worth of bonds—enough to buy eight planes. The first was named after the state association; others were named after the state districts, the Arkansas Drug Travelers,* and the Arkansas Druggists Women's Auxiliary.[26] According to a preliminary tally, the drive sold enough bonds to purchase fifty-four ambulance planes; Wisconsin alone paid for nine.[27]

The results of the 4th War Loan Drive were so positive that a similar approach was used by some state associations during the 5th War Loan Drive, June 12 to July 8, 1944. The objective this time was the purchase of an ambulance train coach. The train was a complete hospital on wheels. It contained treatment areas, a surgical suite, a pharmacy, and nurses' quarters as well as coaches for the wounded. The coaches cost $81,250 in "E" bonds. Unlike the ambulance planes, there were no naming opportunities, but plaques honoring the sponsor would be placed in each coach.[28] The New York City pharmacists raised over $3 million of bond sales to purchase a train that would stretch over a half mile.[29] The trains picked up returning wounded soldiers from ships on either coast. The train would then move inland, depositing the soldiers at hospitals and bases as close to their hometowns as possible. Jack Rodda, a 1935 pharmacy graduate of the University of California, was an Army officer eventually assigned to riding these trains. His train would start at one coast and finish at the other, and then turn around and repeat the trip.[30]

Drug travelers was a term used to identify all of the salesmen who called on drugstores. This included manufacturers' representatives as well as those from wholesalers and other suppliers. Most state associations had a travelers section.

There were other opportunities for pharmacists to raise funds for a particular project. For example, the Washington State Pharmaceutical Association and the King County (Seattle area) Retail Druggists' Association sponsored a LST (landing ship, tank) at its commissioning and provided a $500 check for recreational equipment. The ship was commanded by James L. Randles Jr., a 1939 graduate of the pharmacy school at the University of Washington.[31]

The U.S. Treasury used retailers as a natural sales outlet in all of the war loan drives; drugstores with their long hours and community presence were an integral part of the effort.[32] Even as late as May 1945, no other retail field surpassed the success of the initial drug trade drive. For example, the North Carolina Pharmaceutical Association stores reported sales of over $8 million through the end of 1944.[33]

CONSERVATION EFFORTS

Conservation efforts for strategic and scarce materials started long before the events of Pearl Harbor. The government stockpile of essential drugs as of December 27, 1941, fell far short of its objective (see Table 4.2).[34]

TIN CONSERVATION

Tin was an essential metal for the war effort. Under the headline "Why Save Tin Cans?" a U.S. Government Printing Office pamphlet emphasized that "tin heals," "tin protects," and "tin fights." The "tin fights" section covered the importance of tin for preventing corrosion and listed the tin requirements of various armaments; each submarine needed more than three tons, each heavy bomber forty-eight pounds, each medium tank thirty-five pounds. The "tin protects" section noted the need for tin as protective covering for food, since almost all food sent overseas was packed in tin. The "tin heals" section stated:

> TIN—100% pure TIN—enclosed the little individual morphine hypodermic syringe (Syrette) which soothes the pain of the soldier lying wounded on the field. TIN encases the emergency sulfa ointments which protect him from deadly infection in the

jungle—which help heal his burns—which relieves injuries to his eyes. TIN safeguards the precious blood plasma which enables the Medical Corps to save countless lives right at the front lines by promptly treating loss of blood, shock, and burns. TIN is used for those medicines, because TIN is the most perfect protective covering. No other metal, or substitute, will serve as well. TIN containers of many kinds are indispensable to every Army and Navy Medical Corps doctor, every ambulance company, and every field and base hospital. Millions of these various TIN items are urgently needed.[35]

The need for tin increased in pace with war production, but the supply was critically short; less than 25 percent of the goal of 207,434 long tons was stockpiled in December 1941. The Japanese controlled 70 percent of the world's production, and the United States received 90 percent of its supply from the enemy-held areas. The only way to get tin was to strictly ration its use and to salvage as much as possible in the United States.*

A program of voluntary tin collection was developed by the War Production Board and the Tin Salvage Institute, a body formed by the Packaging Institute of America and the Collapsible Tube Manufacturers' Association. The salvage effort was announced in early January 1942 with radio spots and posters. Initially the public was asked to save their tubes and await later instructions. When the collection plan was developed, the advertisements were changed and the public was told to take the tubes to a drugstore. The Tin Salvage Institute estimated that there were more than 6,000 tons of tin in distribution as tubes; that 85 percent of all tin collapsible tubes were used in drugstore products; and that twenty to twenty-five tons of tin tubes were thrown out daily.[36]

Drugstores were encouraged to provide deposit bins for customers' used tubes. A collection bin placard was developed and, along with an accompanying window banner, was distributed to all drug-

---

*The largest tin smelting operation in the Western world was in Holland; there was no tin smelting operation in the United States. Most of the ore came from the Dutch East Indies, with China, the Belgian Congo, and Bolivia producing smaller amounts. Jones, J. H. with Angly, E. (1951). *Fifty Billion Dollars: My Thirteen Years with the RFC (1932-1945)*. New York: The Macmillan Company, pp. 434-439.

TABLE 4.2. Shortages of Critical Medicines

Drugs	Objective	Percentage on Hand	Medicinal Use
Aconite root	50,000 pounds	0	Powerful poison used to quiet the overaction of the heart. Most imports came from Germany and Spain.
Belladonna leaves and roots	200,000 pounds 60,000 pounds	0	Potent poison, the active ingredient is atropine used to check secretions, stimulate circulation, stimulate respiration, and overcome spasms of involuntary muscles. Major sources were Central Europe and England.
Ergot of rye	200,000 pounds	31	Stimulant for involuntary muscles including the heart and blood vessels. Used to treat shock and migraines. Major sources included Russia, Germany, and Spain.
Henbane leaves	100,000 pounds	0	Antispasmodic action similar to belladonna. Europe was a leading source.
Quinine	9,200,000 avoirdupois ounces	84	Used to treat malarial fevers. Primary source was the Dutch East Indies.
Red squill	675,000 pounds	0	Slows and strengthens the pulse and contracts the blood vessels. Major sources were the European countries bordering on the Mediterranean.
Santonin	1,000 pounds	0	Used primarily as a vermifuge. Major supply was the Orient.

Source: Wood, H. C., LaWall, C. H., Younken, H. W., Osol, A., Griffith, I., and Gershenfeld, L. (1937). *The Dispensatory of the United States of America,* Twenty-Second Edition. Philadelphia: J.B. Lippincott.

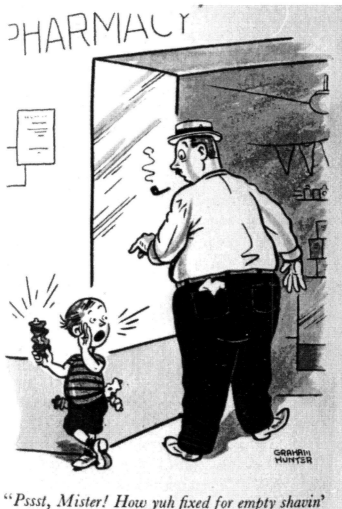

"Pssst, Mister! How yuh fixed for empty shavin' cream tubes?"

The Tin Salvage Institute estimated that 85 percent of all tin collapsible tubes were used in drugstore products, and that twenty to twenty-five tons of tin tubes were thrown out daily. The tin conservation program required that an empty tube had to be turned in when a new tube of shaving cream or toothpaste was purchased. (*Source: Tile and Till* [1942] 28:96. Reprinted with permission of Eli Lilly. Photo courtesy of the Lloyd Library and Museum.)

stores. The banner and placard proclaimed that the drugstore was an "official tin salvage station." Wholesalers agreed to pick up the tubes from their customers when they made their deliveries. Wholesalers were instructed to accumulate tubes in 100-pound lots before sending the tubes, freight collect, to the Tin Salvage Institute in Hillside, New Jersey, for smelting. In localities where wholesalers did not make deliveries, retailers were told to collect tubes in five-pound packages and ship them collect to their wholesaler. Over one-third of 1 million pounds of tubes had been collected by the end of March 1942.

The War Production Board ordered reduced use of tin in civilian packaging and required that a tin tube be exchanged for each new toothpaste or shaving cream tube purchased. The order established three classes of packaging (see Box 4.1). The War Production Board estimated that this step would reduce the use of tin by 4,400 pounds

---

BOX 4.1. Tin Conservation Order

Class I Tubes (100% Tin)

1. Medicinal and pharmaceutical ointments and other preparations extemporaneously compounded or dispensed in manufactured form by pharmacists on legally constituted prescriptions of physicians, dentists, or veterinarians.
2. Ointments and other preparations for ophthalmic use.
3. Solutions for hypodermic injections.
4. Sulfonamide ointment and blood plasma.
5. Diagnostic extracts (allergens).
6. Pile pipes.

Class II Tubes (7 ½% Tin)

1. (a) medicinal and pharmaceutical ointments not included in Class I; (b) preparations which are intended for introduction into body orifices (nasal, vaginal, rectal, surgical jelly, etc.), not included in Class I.

Class III Tubes (7 ½% Tin)

1. Dental cleansing preparations.
2. Shaving preparations.

Source: Title 32, Chapter IX—War Production Board Subchapter B—Division of Industry Operations Post 1147: CollapsableTin, Tin-Coated, and Alloy Tubes Conservation Order M-115. April 2, 1942.

---

during the remainder of 1942.[37] The collection mechanism that had been set up for the voluntary collection was continued.

Between April 1 and September 30, 1942, over 1.168 million pounds of tubes were sent to the Tin Salvage Institute for reclamation. These tubes yielded over 510,000 pounds of tin, most of which were allocated to the war industries. Even a few tubes helped the war effort; sixty tubes provided enough tin to solder all of the connections in a fighter aircraft while 240 tubes would do the job in a heavy bomber.[38] The tin from one salvaged tin can was enough to produce a tube for the morphine Syrette.[39] By the end of 1943 over 7.3 million pounds of tubes had been reclaimed. These yielded almost 1.2 million pounds of tin and 1.5 million pounds of lead.[40]

While toothpaste and shaving cream could still be supplied in tubes, the amount of tubes that could be used was no more than had been sold in 1940. The alternative was to shift sales of dentifrices from toothpaste to tooth powders. Tooth powders that had previously been sold in metal cans were put into new packages made from paper and plastic. Shaving cream manufacturers substituted glass jars for tubes. Many other products had been packaged in metal. Many of the "wets and drys" of the drugstore—products like Epsom salts for consumer sales and milk sugar for use in compounding prescriptions—were quickly repacked into paper containers. The term "Wartime Conservation Container" began to appear on labels, and manufacturers advertised the changed appearance of their products as part of supporting the war effort. For example, Bristol Myers advertised the conversion of its Ingram Shaving Cream noting that Uncle Sam needed the lead for bullets, and civilians would have to do without tubes.[41] Squibb noted in an advertisement that the packaging changes in its consumer products had already saved over a million pounds of tinplate by February 1943.[42]

The tubes sent to the Tin Salvage Institute were sorted and melted. Ingots of the reclaimed metals were sold to war industries for use in essential products. The price to the manufacturers was enough to recover all costs of the operation, and profits were turned over to the Metals Reserve Company,* a subsidiary of the Reconstruction Fi-

---

*Established by the Reconstruction Finance Corporation Act of 1933 with the power to produce, procure, and store strategic and critical materials. *Industrial Mobilization for War: History of the War Production Board and Predecessor Agencies 1940-1945.* Volume 1: *Program and Administration.* Washington DC: GPO, 1947. Reprinted by Greenwood Press, New York, 1969, p. 73.

nance Corporation.[43] Some of the tin came back in products that were essential to the health care of the military. Blood plasma was packed in glass that was then inserted into tin cans. The tin offered protection from environmental problems as well as breakage from the rough handling expected in combat conditions.

THE QUININE POOL

A note in the 1940 *Journal of the American Pharmaceutical Association* updated the condition of the Dutch quinine industry after the Nazi occupation of Holland on May 14, 1940. On May 14 the management of the industry was transferred to Bandoeng, Java, part of the Dutch East Indies. Production was to continue at the Bandoengsche Kininefabriek, the largest quinine factory in the world, and ample production was assured with no danger of a shortage.[44] By December 31, 1941, the federal government had stockpiled more than 7.5 million avoirdupois ounces of quinine, 84 percent of the desired 9.2 million avoirdupois ounces; their stockpile going into 1942 would have to suffice until the source could be regained or adequate alternatives put into place. Then, in March 1942, Java fell to invading Japanese troops and the world supply of quinine was lost to America and her allies.

Malaria was a significant problem. In the United States alone over 4 million cases of malaria were reported in 1937.[45] The disease was endemic in the southern and southeastern regions of the country, areas that would become home to many military training facilities as the war progressed. Of more concern, however, was that all of the war theaters—North Africa, China-Burma-India, Europe, and the Pacific—were in malarial areas.

Malaria is caused by a species of *Plasmodium,* a parasite carried by the female *Anopheles* mosquito. The parasite multiplies in the red blood cells of a host; when the cells rupture, breakdown products cause cycles of chills, fever, and sweating. The combination of effects is devastating to troops in the field, especially in combat conditions.

Quinine was the only medicine that was effective in both preventing and treating malaria. It was also used to treat a number of other medical conditions that ranged from inevitable abortion (a pregnancy in which cramping and bleeding cannot be stopped) to varicose veins (see Box 4.2). Quinine was also used in many proprietary cold and fe-

Stores donated their quinine to the national quinine pool. After the contribution was recorded, the War Production Board acknowledged the gift with an orange "V" certificate. Store owners were instructed to hang the acknowledgment in a public place, such as by their licenses, making the public aware of the contribution. (*Source:* Photo reprinted with permission of the Marvin Samson Center for the History of Pharmacy at University of the Sciences in Philadelphia.)

ver products of the period and as an essential ingredient in products such as sunburn preventatives, hair tonics, and bitter tonics.

On April 4, 1942, the War Production Board issued Conservation Order M-131 to establish control over the supply and distribution of quinine. The order applied to manufacturers, wholesalers, and retailers who had more than fifty ounces of quinine or fifty pounds of cinchona bark on hand. Quinine was restricted to use as an antimalarial agent and in combination with urea hydrochloride for hypodermic use. The National Formulary (NF) Committee immediately noted that the order would affect at least six NF preparations—Elixir of Cinchona Alkaloids; Elixir of Iron, Quinine, and Strychnine; Elixir of Iron, Quinine, and Strychnine Phosphates; Compound Elixir of Glycerophosphates; Compound Syrup of Hypophosphates; and Pills of Iron, Quinine, Strychnine, and Arsenic. The purpose of the NF action was to seek replacements for quinine or remove it altogether and

---

BOX 4.2. Quinine Therapeutics

Abortion (inevitable)
Abscess
Alcoholism
Alopecia
Anemia
Anorexia
Auricular fibrillation
Carbuncle
Conjunctivitis (pneumococcic)
Coronary occlusion
Coryza
Dysentery (amoebic)
Empyema (pneumococcic) in infants and children
Erysipelas
Erythema nodosum
Goiter (exophthalmic)
Hay fever
Hemorrhoids
Herpes zoster (shingles)
Herpes zoster ophthalmicus

Influenza
Local anesthesia (with urea hydrochloride)
Lumbago
Lupus erythematosus
Malaria
Meningitis (pneumococcic)
Paroxysmal tachycardia
Pemphigus
Pertussis (whooping cough)
Pneumonia (lobar)
Psoriasis
Puerperal infection
Sepsis
Typhoid fever
Typhus fever
Ulcer of cornea (pneumococcic)
Uterine inertia (during first stage of labor)
Varicose veins

Source: Quinine Formulary, Merk & Co., Rahway, NJ, 1933.

rename the product.[46] On April 30, 1942, Order M-131 was amended to include totaquine, a mixture of cinchona alkaloids. The National Formulary Committee encouraged pharmacists to return full, unopened packages of quinine and totaquine to their suppliers as a patriotic gesture. A new monograph was issued for Elixir of Iron and Strychnine with the quinine removed.[47] On June 19, the War Production Board issued a modified Conservation Order, M-131a, to include cinchonine, cinchonidine, and quinidine and reduce the exemption of quinine from fifty ounces to ten ounces. The use of quinine, cinchonine, and cinchonidine was restricted to malaria; quinidine was restricted to use only in malaria or cardiac disorders.[48]

The quinine conservation orders, M-131 and M-131a, virtually froze quinine use in the drugstore prescription area. Legally, the only time that quinine could be used was for malaria, and in many areas there was no malaria. On July 1, 1942, a survey of 1,800 retail New Jersey drugstores reported over 3,700 packages (over 3,500 ounces) of cinchona alkaloids in original containers.[49] In September, Ivor Griffith, dean of the Philadelphia College of Pharmacy, contacted the War Production Board and offered to collect, identify, and assay quinine from alumni and later from all drugstores in Pennsylvania. The college forwarded the materials without charge to the Defense Supplies Corporation for military use.* By December, almost 1,000 donors had forwarded over 11,000 packages of different compounds and dose forms, between 6,000 and 8,000 ounces of quinine. The experiment was a success; in January, the quinine collection went national.[50]

The War Production Board and the Defense Supplies Corporation authorized the American Pharmaceutical Association, as an agent of the government, to establish a national quinine pool in the basement of the headquarters building.[51] A special appeal asking pharmacists to donate the quinine from their shelves was developed, and a six-page flyer was sent to every drugstore in the country. The flyer included personal appeals from Ross McIntyre, the surgeon general of

---

*Established by the Reconstruction Finance Corporation Act of 1933 with the power to produce, procure, and store strategic and critical materials. *Industrial Mobilization for War: History of the War Production Board and Predecessor Agencies 1940-1945.* Volume 1: *Program and Administration.* Washington, DC: GPO, 1947. Reprinted by Greenwood Press, New York, 1969, p. 73.

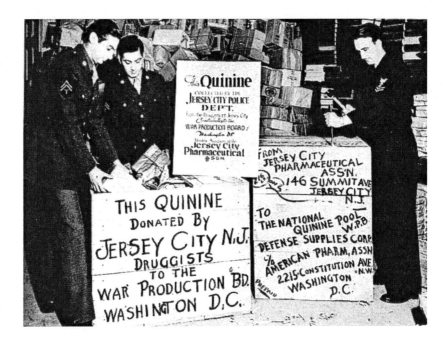

There was an immediate response to the announcement that quinine sitting on store shelves could be turned in to help the war effort. In many cases the state and local associations coordinated the drive to increase participation. Stores, colleges, and wholesalers forwarded opened and unopened bottles of quinine to the national quinine pool, which was located in the lower level of the American Pharmaceutical Association building. (*Source: New Jersey Journal of Pharmacy* [1943] 16: cover. Reprinted with permission. Photo courtesy of the Lloyd Library and Museum.)

the Navy, and Larry McAfee, the acting surgeon general of the Army, recounting the importance of quinine for the military and the support that pharmacists could provide by donating it.

A process for receiving, recording, and sorting quinine was established, and staff were assigned to the quinine pool. Contributions were opened and the contents logged, along with the name and address of the contributor. The contents were sorted according to the salt and the dose form, and opened packages were combined into large drums. Each contribution was acknowledged with a "V" Certificate to display as an indication of participation in the war effort.[52]

Many of the contributions were small. For example, in July 619 packages averaging 6.9 ounces per package were opened. However, the collective value was large. During a facility inspection by the secretary of commerce it was noted that several barrels of powders and tablets awaiting shipment to a processor had a pre–Pearl Harbor value of $90,000; the current value was $9 million. One shipment of a dozen barrels of quinine powders was sufficient to supply the entire November 1942 North African invasion force.[53]

Pharmacists responded enthusiastically to the quinine collection. Many state and local associations organized drives and canvassed their members in store-to-store campaigns. The member colleges of the American Association of Colleges of Pharmacy offered their facilities to the War Production Board to assemble their state collections.[54] The trade press told and retold of the need for quinine and the opportunity for pharmacists to make a difference. In North Carolina the governor detailed the state highway patrol to visit every drugstore to collect quinine. Over 8,000 separate bottles totaling 960,407 grains of quinine were collected from two health departments, thirty-four hospitals, and 739 drugstores and physicians' offices. The state board of health was the largest contributor (90,000 grains). The North Carolina Pharmaceutical Association coordinated the drive, sorted the contributions, and forwarded the total to the national quinine pool.[55] Many colleges of pharmacy stripped their central stores and dispensing labs of quinine. In February, Ohio State University forwarded 1,000 five-grain capsules along with 554 grams of quinine sulfate, and forty-five grams of quinine hydrochloride.[56]

The *Journal of the American Medical Association* also published articles supporting the efforts of pharmacists' collections.[57] The quinine drive was featured on national radio to inform the American public about the need for quinine and the involvement of pharmacists in helping to meet that need. The publicity also brought contributions from other, unexpected sources. In Oregon the governor asked citizens to check their medicine cabinets and turn in any quinine to their local druggist for donation to the national pool.[58] A manufacturer of soft drinks found in storage some quinine from a discontinued tonic. The Home of the Aged and Infirm in Washington, DC, discovered 9,000 three-grain quinine pills that had been in storage since the end of World War I.[59] Even President Roosevelt participated, by contributing 110 pounds of quinine sulfate that he had received as a gift from the president of Peru.[60] Since quinine does not deteriorate with age, all of these contributions were welcomed and added to the quinine pool.

The quinine drive was concluded and the operations of the pool discontinued in October 1942. The original goal for the operation was 100,000 ounces of quinine. The final accounting of the campaign showed the success of the effort. In the nine months that the quinine pool had been in operation, over 17,000 shipments had been logged. The total amount of quinine collected was in excess of 150,000 ounces (more than 6.5 million ten-grain doses).[61] This was in addition to the 1,300 packages (12,000 ounces) of quinine gathered by the Philadelphia College of Pharmacy in 1942.[62]

The quinine collected during the drive was an important war contribution. The only other antimalarial of any value in the combat areas was Atabrine; many troops refused to take it because its side effects of nausea, vomiting, and headaches were as bad as the symptoms of malaria. Some of the early research into absorption, metabolism, and excretion patterns was undertaken to find an answer to the problem. This new way of looking at how medicines worked in the body was the beginnings of clinical pharmacology. By the spring of 1943 the toxicity problem was solved by providing a loading dose followed by the daily administration of a maintenance dose.[63]

COMMUNITY SERVICE

In his 1944 message on National Pharmacy Week, APhA President George Moulton addressed the community services that pharmacies and pharmacists were making to the war effort. He noted some of the highlights, such as more prescriptions being filled than ever before, the successful quinine drive, the improvised and new products emerging from the manufacturers, and the ability to meet almost every need for essential medicines. He emphasized that all advances were composed of the efforts of thousands of individuals, not just the few who made the headlines. He noted the need to make it obvious to the public that

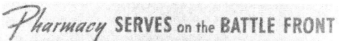

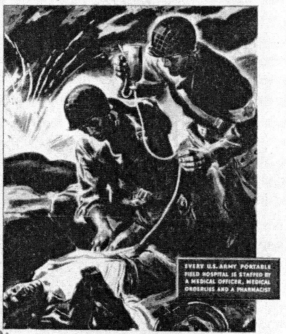

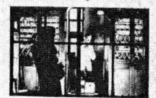

A number of companies produced ads saluting pharmacy's role in the war effort at home and in the Armed Forces. These would frequently be produced as counter cards and distributed through wholesalers for display in the drugstore. McKesson's ad details the health care role of pharmacy and the education required to compound the "most intricate" of prescriptions. (*Source: Northwestern Druggist* [1945]53 [February]:36. Photo courtesy of Lloyd Library and Museum.)

pharmacists were not just drug merchants, that they were practicing a profession that embraced service to humanity.[64]

Historian Michael Flannery described the centrality of the drugstore as an integral part of the social fabric of the community and then added "as an arsenal of ever-expanding therapeutic armamentarium, the drugstore became the most convenient ally in the struggle against the ravages of disease; only the church offered a more potent promise of relief."[65]

Less obvious to the public and with little acclaim was the kind of personal community service provided by the local pharmacist. A sad illustration of this is recounted by Douglas D. Glover, the son of Douglas Glover. The senior Glover graduated from the University of Maryland in 1913 and served in the Army during World War I. After the war he moved to the small town of Rowlesburg, West Virginia (population 1,500), where he operated the only drugstore. Young Glover remembered:

> Small communities had limited, if any, telephone service, and few small towns had access to a Western Union office. Telegrams were transmitted over the B&O wires and received by the railroad telegrapher. Glover's Drugstore had one of about thirty telephones in town. Upon receipt of a telegram the telegrapher would call my father and dictate the telegram. As clerk, it was my job to deliver the handwritten telegram by bicycle. As our armed forces became engaged in combat it was inevitable that casualties would follow. Next of kin were notified by telegram when a serviceman was killed or wounded in action. Upon receipt of a telegram beginning with "The Secretary of War regrets to inform you . . ." my father would personally deliver the dreadful news. Each event was individualized, and considerable thought was given as to how the emotional impact of the message could be minimized.[66]

Chapter 5

Pharmacy Operations

The war years beginning in January 1942 and ending in December 1945 were not a homogenous period. The retail world in general was not the same in 1941 or 1942 as it was in late 1944 and 1945. The opening months of 1942 did not yet have the rationing and shortages of some items that would occur later. The population had not yet sent almost 12 million men into uniform. The mass migration from rural America into the cities and industries of wartime production had not yet occurred. Rosie the Riveter, representing more than 5 million women who left the traditional role of housewife and entered the workforce after the declaration of war, had not yet taken her place in the workplace. Men would go to work in the war industries or enter the armed forces. Wages would climb higher than they had ever been before. Rationing would arrive, mostly to save critical materials for war industries but also to control distribution, ensuring that everyone had equal access to items in short supply. The federal government would establish price controls to control inflation. Retail pharmacy would be part of the World War II changes.[1]

SHORTAGES AND RATIONING

At the beginning of the war, drugstore owners were unsure about their financial future. Articles in the trade press cautioned pharmacists to prepare for difficult operating conditions.[2,3] Even before America entered the war there had been a growing awareness of looming shortages of essential medicines. In January 1941 Joseph A. Hailer, manager of the Pharmaceutical Department at United Drug, wrote to the field sales representatives servicing the company's retail stores (United Drug, Owl Drug, and Liggett Drug) and Rexall agency stores. He stated that United had a good supply of products so their stores would experience fewer restrictions than other stores with different wholesalers and suppliers.[4] Early in 1941 exports of belladonna and atropine were restricted in the interest of national defense;[5] by October, there were concerns over the ability to obtain "papaws," as papayas were known, which were the source for papain that was used for the debridement of necrotic tissue.[6] A foretaste of handling shortages by changing official standards occurred in October as the shortage of ergot became evident. Domestic production was in short supply, and the normal sources in Spain were unable to gain airtight containers to ship their ergot to the United States. The issue with the Spanish source was that the amount of moisture in the product was in excess of USP standards. The suggested solution was to permit a temporary waiver on the moisture content in order to get the ergot shipped quickly and then remove the excess moisture once it arrived in the States.[7]

The National Formulary Committee devised substitutes and formulation changes. Cudbear was the approved coloring agent for ten NF preparations, but imports from war areas had ceased. The NF Committee allowed amaranth solution as a substitute coloring agent in these formulas. Similarly, oil of bitter almond, a flavoring agent, was also in scarce supply. The NF Council approved substitution of Benzaldehyde NF as the flavoring agent in NF preparations. Manufacturers of Hinkle's Pills, a cathartic, requested that they be allowed to use extract of stramonium in place of extract of belladonna. Stramonium was plentiful and had the same activity of the rapidly disappearing belladonna.[8]

In May 1942, the New York Academy of Medicine established a subcommittee to investigate war shortages of essential medicines and appliances. The subcommittee was chaired by Walter Bastedo, a pharmacist and physician who was serving as the president of the United States Pharmacopoeia.[9] The subcommittee's report identified the competing needs of the armed forces, Lend-Lease, and civilians for medicines in light of the present and anticipated shortages, either because of the loss of supply from abroad or because of increased military needs. The military had reportedly ordered 100,000 vials of tetanus antitoxin, 40 million quinine tablets, 35 million sulfathiazole tablets, and 10 million sulfapyradine tablets. The sulfas alone repre-

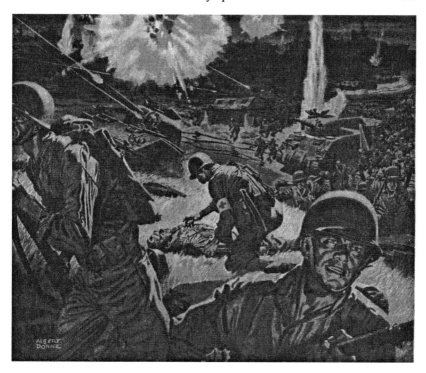

"Just a Pill-Roller from Paducah?...Listen..."

"WE'RE TOUGH, our outfit is. Tough as nails, and our record proves it. But that doesn't mean we're not willing to eat our words about something. ...You see, it's about that little pill-roller from Paducah...

"Back in the States, training, we didn't think any outfit came up to ours. And were we fancy with the big talk! Especially when it was about the pill-rollers. You know, the Army medics...

"Hey, this here pill-roller is from Paducah. Isn't he cute?"

"Root-de-toot for the bedpan battalion."

"Then we went overseas. And it was the big boss himself who picked us to go in first and grab the beachhead. You read about it in the papers, I guess.

"It was hell, plain hell. We beached under heavy fire. The sky looked like a crazy Fourth of July as we poured out of the barges. Guys dropped right and left alongside me. I didn't have time to do much looking around — but I did see Paducah and the other pill-rollers.

"They were right with us, every inch of the way ... caring for guys as they fell ... calmly doing their jobs right out there in the open with all hell busted loose.

"Well, there isn't much more we can say. There just aren't words. But, if you ever hear anybody talking about pill-rollers in a smart-aleck kind of way ... just tell them to talk to a guy who has seen some action. He'll set 'em straight on pill-rollers. But fast!"

A tribute to the members of the

U. S. ARMY MEDICAL DEPT.

By the world's largest makers of surgical dressings

Johnson-Johnson

Many of the companies kept their names in front of the public through advertising the military. Johnson & Johnson developed a series of ads featuring the U.S. Army Medical Department. This example offers a tribute to the Army's pillrollers.

sented the civilian needs of the entire country for two or three months. Chemicals needed for the production of medicines were being requested for use in war production, especially alcohol, phenol, glycerin, and potassium. While alcohol was essential for manufacturing ether, insulin, and tinctures, it was a critical ingredient in smokeless gunpowder. It took sixty-five gallons of alcohol to make every sixteen-inch artillery shell. Supplying the medical needs of America's allies was also a high priority. Britain looked to America for all its insulin, since Britain's manufacturers had been demolished in the bombing. The report noted that the U.S. Pharmacopoeia and others were developing standards for efficient substitutes and that civilian needs were also a priority of the War Production Board. Physicians were urged to be prudent in their use of medicines and limit scarce items to situations in which no appropriate substitutes were available. Physicians were also urged to find alternatives for liquid preparations containing glycerin and alcohol and to use sodium salts in preference to potassium.[10]

In May, Justin Powers, the director of the National Formulary and the newly appointed editor of the *Journal of the American Pharmaceutical Association,* Scientific Edition, addressed the annual meeting of the American Drug Manufacturers Association on war problems. He discussed the possibility of a war formulary which would either require or allow the discontinuation of products with unavailable ingredients. However, the general sentiment of both the USP and NF advisors was that substitutions could be made in most cases without sacrificing the quality of the product. Powers, noting the earlier action on both the Elixir of Cudbear and Oil of Bitter Almond, added that many ingredients (such as Orange Flower Water and Oil of Dwarf Pine Needles) could simply be eliminated without jeopardizing the medicinal value of the product. Shipments of Arnica had become a problem, but some indigenous species of Arnica could be substituted without fear of violation of the Food, Drug, and Cosmetic Act. Alcohol continued to be a problem because it was a critical war materiel. A suggestion to substitute wine was being explored, but the Bureau of Internal Revenue had taken the position that viniferous products must contain 45 percent medicinal solids to make them unpalatable.[11] Within the first five months after America's entry into the war a list of shortages for the manufacture of medicines was already over 200 items. The most pressing items, in addition to quinine, are listed in Box 5.1. The shortages of alcohol, sugar, and glycerin accelerated the movement from liquid dosage forms to dry oral dosage forms.[12]

By late 1942 glycerin, a common pharmaceutical solvent, was becoming increasingly difficult to obtain for use in pharmaceutical products. By official definition, elixirs were required to contain glycerin and many National Formulary galenicals also used glycerin. The APhA laboratory announced in early 1943 that glycerin could be reduced in the official elixirs and reduced or eliminated in other formulations without affecting appearance or effectiveness. In many cases liquid glucose could be substituted for the glycerin.[14]

Sugar restrictions, imposed in January 1942, provided a challenge for both retail pharmacists and manufacturers. In prescription practice sugar was an essential ingredient in compounding; it was also important in the operation of fountains and lunch counters. For exam-

---

BOX 5.1. Shortages in 1942[13]

Acetic acid	Citric acid	Oil, almond
Acetone	Creasote	Oil, cardamon
Agar	Ethyl cellulose	Oil, cassia
Albumin	Eucalyptol	Oil, castor
Alcohol, benzyl	Formaldehyde	Oil, cinnamon
Alcohol, ethyl	Glycerin	Oil, citronella
Alcohol, isopropyl	Guaiacol	Oil, cloves
Alcohol, methyl	Gum arabic	Oil, olive
Aminophylline	Henbane	Oil, pine needles
Ammonia and its salts	Hexamethylenetetramine	Phenol and its derivatives
Ascorbic acid	Hycosine	Potassium salts
Atropine	Hypochlorites	Salicylates
Belladonna	Lanolin	Sodium benzoate
Benzaldehyde	Licorice	Sodium perborate
Benzyl esters	Liver extract	Sugar
Brucine	Magnesium and its salts	Theobromine
Caffeine		Thymol
Chlorbutanol	Menthol	Triethanolamine
Chlorinated hydrocarbons	Mercury and its salts	Vitamin A
Chlorine	Metallic salts	Zinc oxide
Chloroform	Nicotinamide	

ple, one Key West drugstore's fountain and lunch counter sales in December of 1942 were over $10,000 and almost 59,000 people were served.[15] However, in late January the Office of Production Management provided retail druggists with documentation allowing them to draw up to ten pounds of sugar a week but only for pharmaceutical and drug uses.[16]

The three most important pharmaceutical solvents, alcohol, glycerin, and sugar, were also essential war product commodities. By 1943 the sugar shortage was an increasing problem for pharmaceutical manufacturers. Supplies were restricted to 70 percent of the 1941 usage. Manufacturers were forced to reduce sugar levels as much as possible while still retaining the product as official under either USP or NF requirements. Some manufacturers sought formulation changes which could mean that the product could no longer be identified as "official." Some products were discontinued, at least for the duration of the war. This led to a concern over label changes and possible confusion for physicians and patients. This was at a period when sugar restrictions were being eased for restaurant and home use.[17]

In May 1942, the Centaur Division of Sterling Drug announced the recall of Fletcher's Castoria, a popular children's laxative.[18] At first it was believed that a foreign ingredient was causing nausea and vomiting, but later investigation showed otherwise. The active ingredient was senna; the original formula included 20 percent sugar. The sugar in the formulation had been reduced several times, seemingly without a problem. However, in April there were changes in the chemical characteristics of the water and this, together with the reduced sugar concentration, altered the fermentation process during manufacturing. After weeks of testing, Centaur announced that Castoria would return to the shelves in a new container with a highlighted control number on each package.[19]

Packaging and closures were also becoming problematic. Tin was in short supply and its use restricted; drugstores collected empty collapsible tubes for recycling. Pharmaceutical manufacturers had to prove that substitute packaging was safe and effective or risk discontinuing their products until either some alternative packaging was available or the war ended. Many products were put into wartime conservation packs of glass, cardboard, or similar paper products. Glass containers became the most common replacement for topical products such as shaving cream and cosmetics. Many manufacturers of proprietary products and toiletries saved packaging materials by discontinuing smaller sizes and thereby reducing the number of product sizes sold. Conversely, manufacturers of prescription medicines also eliminated some product sizes but maintained the smaller sizes to eliminate the amount of unused product and packaging sitting in the consumer's medicine cabinet or on the drugstore shelf.[20]

Shortages removed many items from drugstore shelves as metals and other materials were prioritized for military use. Small items, such as hair pins, as well as clocks, watches, flashlights, batteries, cameras, heating pads, and similar merchandise became almost impossible for retailers to obtain. Rubber goods, such as hot water bottles and fountain syringes, disappeared. Manufacturers used their advertising space to inform consumers on how to keep an old product in good working order or that the product had "gone to war" for the duration. Wrigley chewing gums completely disappeared as the military took the total production for its use. Wrigley ran advertisements suggesting that its chewing gums were making the lives of soldiers, sailors, marines, and airmen in combat more bearable. Jack Olson recalled his father's drugstore on the corner of Hollywood and Wilton in Los Angeles. At the beginning of the war there was a rumor of an impending shortage of Kotex and Modess and so it would be a good idea to stock up, "and stock up he did, cases in the storage area and in the garage at home. Really prepared, right? Wrong! There was a shortage of toilet paper instead."[21]

Wartime conditions did not create as many problems for drugstores as for other retailers. Drugstore owners experienced fewer merchandise shortages than other retailers and only a portion of their merchandise was subject to rationing.[22] An executive of McKesson and Robbins, a large drug wholesaler of the period, advised druggists not to worry about selling things that you cannot get, "but to do everything possible to get more business with the things that you can get."[23] Sales volume lost due to these shortages was more than made up by increased sales of health items. At least some felt that the drugstore was once again becoming a pharmacy.[24] Herman Mueller, secretary of the National Guild of Hy-Pure Druggists, a buying group of 400 independent druggists, suggested that a long war would result in drugstores becoming more professional and less cluttered with the

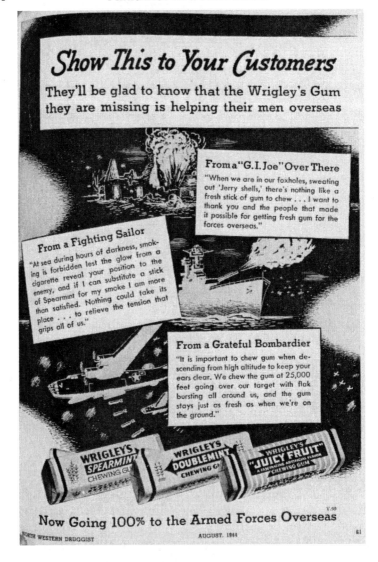

Many products were in short supply and some items completely disappeared. Manufacturers explained that their products had gone to war in advertising designed to keep the product in the buying public's memory for after the war. Wrigley's Gum was included in military rations and was not available at civilian candy counters. (*Source: Northwestern Druggist* [1944] 52:61. Photo courtesy of the Lloyd Library and Museum.)

convenience merchandise that made up a large part of the drugstore in 1942.[25]

Drugstore fountains were particularly affected by the shortages of sugar and other foodstuffs. As an example, ice cream was in short supply in most parts of the country. Dairies were forced to curtail delivery schedules, and milk products had a limited shelf life. Sugar, meat, and other foodstuffs were rationed, and many of the packaging materials were not available. Perhaps the greatest challenge to the fountain, however, was the shortage of manpower. Most of the boys and young men who had been employed as "soda jerks" were in the military or working in higher-paying jobs in war plants. There were no new fountains produced, replacement parts were scarce, and fountain gases were essential war materials. The *NARD Wartime Guide* suggested many alternatives for drugstore owners to maintain their fountain operation, including utilizing more women, maintaining equipment better, using self-service items, and closing the fountain earlier.[26] Many store owners, unable to find alternative supplies and personnel, closed their fountains for the duration. Jo Biemesderfer, writing about ice cream shortages in her father's Lansdale, Pennsylvania, drugstore, recalled that sugar rationing put a halt to homemade fountain syrups and chocolate syrup was not available because of the lack of the dark cocoa from the East Indies. Whenever an ice cream flavor was shorted or discontinued, her father would post a hand-printed sign "D . . . that Hitler, we are out of (whatever flavor) again!"[27]

JAPANESE AMERICANS

There were other reasons that stores were forced to close as a consequence of the war. In 1942, due to Executive Order 9066, individuals of Japanese descent were forcibly removed from California and the western parts of Washington and Oregon. In May 1942 it was estimated that as many as twenty-five drugstores operated by Japanese Americans in the Los Angeles area were forced to close.[28] Drugstore owners were forced to quickly dispose of their belongings and businesses, frequently at a heavy financial loss. One estimate of the property that had to be left behind was at least $200 million.[29] Sam Kitabayashi was a 1939 graduate of the University of San Francisco.

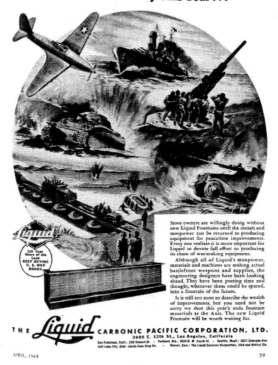

The soda fountain was an important part of many drugstores before the war. Many stores closed their fountains
because of rationing, especially of sugar and syrups, and
the lack of men to operate them. The Liquid Carbonic Pacific Corporation explained what was happening to its production of fountains and added that its designers were
already thinking about the "fountain of the future." (*Source:
Pacific Drug Review* [1943] 55:39. Photo courtesy of the
Lloyd Library and Museum.)

He worked in retail pharmacy from graduation until early 1941 when
he opened his own store. He recalled that he

> never served in the armed forces of the U.S. or the Merchant
> Marines—but I did practice in the retail trade until mid-May
> 1942. Being of Japanese descent, although a U.S. citizen, we

had to give up everything and I was sent to Heart Mountain, Wyoming Relocation Center from 1942 to 1945.[30]

George Tokuda graduated from the University of Washington. Like many other Nisei he understood that one way to avoid discrimination was to do something on his own. After graduation he bought a store in Seattle and later started a second. His wife remembered:

> When George faced evacuation, he consolidated his merchandise into his original drugstore and stored the fixtures of store number two. Not knowing how long he would be gone, he asked a Caucasian neighbor to maintain his business. When he was in Camp Harmony [Puyallup, Washington], a friend came to tell him that the store was almost empty. During that time George had received less than one hundred dollars from the caretaker. He requested camp authorities if he could be granted a one-day leave to Seattle, but permission was not granted. He made contact with a Seattle lawyer and had him sell what was left, fixtures and all, for $1,900. Of that, $400 went to the attorney. When he returned to Seattle, in 1945, he discovered the man to whom he had sold the store had put up a sign, "No Japs."[31]

Japanese Americans were moved first to assembly areas and later to one of ten relocation camps away from the West Coast (see Chapter 2). In a survey of the camps taken in November 1942, at least ninety-six pharmacists were already interred.[32] Some were allowed to work as pharmacists in the camps or were given duties in the hospitals or clinics as technicians. In some cases the Japanese American pharmacists could avoid the camps through relocation away from the coastal areas. This available manpower was not ignored. At the regular meeting of the Michigan Board of Pharmacy on June 19, 1944, reciprocity was granted to John Yoshio Furuta from Washington State who was classified by his draft board as 4-F, unable to serve for medical reasons. At the same meeting the board voted to allow Miss Takaye Fukuhara, a graduate of the University of California and registered in California, to take the state board the next day.[33]

Reciprocity was a problem for those who managed to avoid the camps or gain release to move inland. Benjamin Matsuda, a University of California—San Francisco graduate, owned a store in Watsonville, California. He voluntarily left before General DeWitt issued Proclamation No. 4 on March 27, 1942, forbidding voluntary migration out of the military areas. He had to quickly pack up and get rid of his stock as best he could before moving to Denver. He was without a Colorado license and ended up working as a farm laborer until he could reciprocate.[34]

ECONOMICS

The drugstore of the early 1940s was a small business that could be found in towns and neighborhoods almost everywhere in America. A majority of the stores had only one pharmacist. The average drugstore was open sixteen hours a day, seven days a week.[35] Data from 1939 break down the sales volume in the average drugstore as follows: cigars and cigarettes, 20 percent; soda fountain, 24 percent; prescriptions and crude drugs, 15 percent; patent medicines, 13 percent; cosmetics, dentifrices, and toiletries, 8 percent; sundries, 6 percent; candy, 5 percent; control line, 3 percent; surgical dressings and hospital supplies, 3 percent; and vitamins, 2 percent.[36] The average price for a compounded prescription in 1940 was ninety-three cents.[37] At the outset of the war, chains accounted for approximately 23 percent of the total volume of the retail drug field but less than 9 percent of the prescription volume.[38] In 1942, *Drug Topics* reported that there were over 60,000 drugstores, 54,912 independents, and 5,276 chain units in the United States.[39]

In spite of problems with shortages and restrictions, the percentage of retail pharmacies operating at a loss during the war years decreased from 9 percent in 1941 to 3 percent in 1945. In the decade of the 1930s, the percentage was in double digits ranging from 34 percent in 1932 to 12 percent in 1935.[40] By January 1943, after only one year of war, approximately 15.5 percent of the drugstores had closed as licensed pharmacies.[41] Massachusetts reported that 10 percent of its stores had closed[42] and in March of 1944 Iowa reported that fifty-five stores had closed in the prior year.[43] The closings were the result of a number of factors. One was the unavailability of pharmacists, which meant that when older men tried to sell their stores and retire, no one was there to buy them. In normal times, young pharmacists opened new stores, which offset stores closed due to the death or retirement of the owner. This was unusual during the war, as fewer men graduated from pharmacy school and many of those who did were soon in the military. The absence of purchasers also affected those owners who went into the military. Some owners were able to sell their stores; some surrendered the pharmacy license but kept the store open without prescription services; and some closed. Phil Teague in Columbus, Ohio, was drafted and had to close his store. His wholesaler accepted all unopened merchandise for credit, and all opened merchandise was transferred to another pharmacist, Howard Eberts, to store or to use if he could.[44]

In 1942 pharmacies were eligible to purchase insurance against losses due to enemy actions or actions of the U.S. armed forces in resisting invasion. This insurance was offered through the War Damage Corporation, a subsidiary of the federal Reconstruction Finance Corporation. All insurance companies were eligible to sell the policies. The policies for business with inventories not used for manufacturing cost $1.40 per $1,000 of insurance at 80 percent coinsurance. Insurance was also available on homes and contents beginning at $1.00 per $1,000 of value.[45] C. W. Bates of Los Angeles purchased a policy through Ohio Farmer's Insurance on July 8, 1942. For the $6,000 policy covering the stock and fixtures of his drugstore he paid $7.20 plus a commission of $1.00.[46]

It was difficult to start a new drugstore during the war years. Even if there was a pharmacist who wanted to do so, new shelving, fountains, and display units were difficult, if not impossible, to obtain.[47] Building materials were prioritized because many common items such as lumber, nails, and fixtures were needed to build the large number of new training facilities and bases, and serve the other needs of the 12-million-strong Armed Forces.

Total retail sales for drugstores increased during the war years. In 1940 the total sales for U.S. drugstores were $1.637 billion and at the end of the war in 1945 the total retail sales were $2.96 billion—an increase of 80 percent. While sales for other retail establishments also increased during the war, the increase was far less.[48] A broad array of factors produced these drugstore sales: more employed people spent more money to stay healthy, and they spent their health care dollars in fewer drugstores.

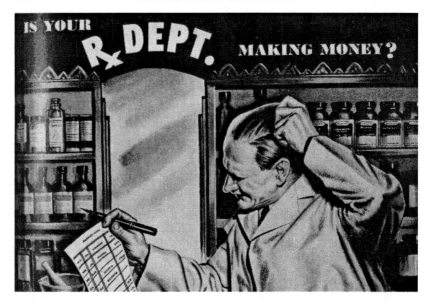

Prescription volume grew from 13.2 percent of total store sales in 1941 to 18.9 percent in 1945. Essential medicines were never rationed during the war years. Physicians were writing more prescriptions and there were fewer stores where they could be filled. Drugstores that operated during the war years did well financially. (*Source: The Apothecary* [1944] 56:125. Photo courtesy of the Lloyd Library and Museum.)

A challenge for consumers was what to buy with these newly earned dollars. New cars, refrigerators, and homes were not available. Clothing, food, and many small consumer goods were rationed. In spite of the absences and shortages, there was plenty to buy.[49] Production for civilian consumption remained high; in 1944, at the height of war production, the total of civilian goods and services was higher than it was in 1940.[50]

A focus on health during the war was perhaps greater than ever before in American life. People had enough money to see and pay a doctor when they were ill. But another factor was at play: it was unpatriotic to be sick. Workers had to stay well to put out their maximum effort to produce. Posters appeared in many war industry plants urging people not to be absent—that such absence helped the enemy. Workers were encouraged to report even minor accidents so that first

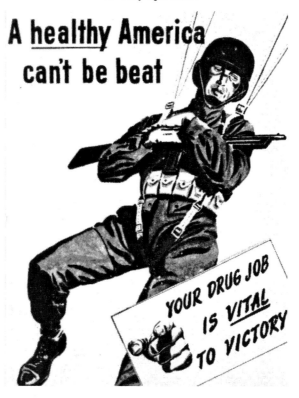

A poster produced by the National Wholesale Druggists' Association was featured on the cover of the *Carolina Journal of Pharmacy* in 1944. It was one of a series designed to ensure "efficient distribution of drugs, medicines, and health supplies so vital to victory." (*Source: Carolina Journal of Pharmacy* [1944] February: cover. Reprinted with permission of the North Carolina Association of Pharmacists. Photo courtesy of the Lloyd Library and Museum.)

aid could be rendered, averting a longer time away from the production work. One example of this fervor was the common toothbrush. Before the war, brushing one's teeth was not the common hygienic task that we appreciate today. Toothbrush manufacturers and others advertised that workers should brush often, thereby avoiding cavities and other health problems that could result in absenteeism and interfere with production. A series of advertisements for Dr. West's toothbrushes quoted Morris Fishbein of the American Medical Association as saying that toothbrushes were essential to national health, yet half of the American population did not even own one. He added "that poor teeth are frequently the underlying cause of poor health. You know . . . we all know that every ounce of productive capacity is needed by our country."[51] Sal Hepatica, a laxative, ran a similar series of advertisements, showing women in war production who could not function at their peak because they felt sluggish due to constipation.[52] For many consumers, the drugstore was the place where they purchased items such as toothbrushes and laxatives.

The drugstore was the single retail outlet that might be identified with the new health consciousness of American purchasers. In the entire war period, medicines were not rationed. The War Production Board had an Office of Civilian Requirements. Robert Fischelis was chief of the Chemicals, Drugs, and Health Supplies Branch. He would become the secretary of the American Pharmaceutical Association in 1945. The chief of the Drugs and Cosmetics Section was Fred Stock, a Purdue graduate, who was a pharmacist with Walgreens before being placed "on loan" with the War Production Board. J. Solon Mordell also served on the staff of the Medical and Health Supplies Section of the War Production Board. In April 1944 the War Production Board set up the Office of Civilian Penicillin Distribution to manage the phased-in distribution of limited stocks of the new miracle drug. John N. McDonnell, a Philadelphia College of Pharmacy graduate before joining the War Production Board, was named to head the office.

A shrinking number of drugstores, the increase in health consciousness, and product availability led to significant sales increases for those drugstores that remained in business. Average sales in the retail pharmacy increased dramatically from approximately $36,000 in 1941 to over $62,000 in 1945. To put this increase into the overall business perspective of all retail stores, during the first six months of 1943 sales in drugstores nationally increased 27 percent over the same period in 1942. The average national sales of all retailers, including drugstores, increased only 17 percent.[53]

In an attempt to better understand the reasons for store closures, the National Wholesale Druggist Association commissioned a Dunn and Bradstreet study. The study was conducted through questionnaires to wholesalers and covered actual closings as well as transfers of ownership. The study did not provide information on individual stores or the total number of closed units, but it noted that loss of pharmacists and clerks accounted for almost half of the closures. In another question, the present occupation of most former proprietors were given: 20 percent were in the military; 20 percent were deceased, ill, or retired; and, 20 percent were working in another pharmacy.[54]

The inventory in drugstores during the war years increased at a rate slightly higher than the increase in sales, especially in 1944. In that year inventory increased 24.6 percent over the previous year compared to an 11.5 percent increase in sales. Increases in inventory were due to several factors, not the least of which was the uncertainty of product delivery or availability. Donald Nelson, head of the War Production Board, encouraged the retailers of health necessities to increase inventories mostly because of difficulties in transportation rather than product shortages, although shortages did occur.[55] In 1943 the War Production Board mandated that sanitary napkins be compressed into packages requiring no more than 13.75 cubic inches, explaining that this would release 2,000 freight cars for shipment of other goods.[56] Drugstore owners bought what they could, whenever they could in this "seller's market."

During the period that sales were increasing, prescription volume was increasing even faster. The latter probably contributed significantly to the former inasmuch as the retail cost of the average prescription was several times as much as the price of other drugstore items.[57] Prescription sales increased from 13.2 percent of total store sales to 19 percent by the end of the war. One report estimated that on average this amounted to an increase of 502 prescriptions per year, almost ten per week.[58] In 1942 physicians wrote an average of 1,266 prescriptions—a 12.7 percent increase over 1941. These increases were in spite of the fact that the civilian population decreased as the military increased in the first year following Pearl Harbor. Patients could pay for their prescriptions out of their increased personal income.[59] Another reason for increased prescriptions being presented to the pharmacist was that many of the physicians who had dispensed medicines from their offices had discontinued the practice. They had difficulty getting materials to dispense, less time to keep up with product availability, and less time due to increased patient load.[60]

On April 28, 1942, the Office of Price Administration placed a maximum price regulation into effect as an anti-inflationary measure. This regulation was designed to freeze prices on a number of goods and services at the March 1942 level. By July each retailer was mandated to post ceiling prices for a list of "Cost of Living Commodities" established by the OPA. Any attempt to sell items for higher prices could result in a fine for both the seller and the buyer. Drugstore products that were listed as cost-of-living commodities included the following:

Tobacco
    Cigarettes
    Smoking tobacco, in cans and packages
Packaged Household Drugs
    Aspirin tablets
    Milk of magnesia, liquid
    Cod liver oil, liquid
    Epsom salts
    Boric acid
    Castor oil and mineral oil
    Witch hazel and rubbing alcohol
Toiletries and sundries
    Hand and toilet soaps
    Dentifrices (paste, powder, and liquid)
    Shaving cream
    Toothbrushes
    Sanitary napkins
    Razor blades
    Facial tissues
Infant foods: all types
Ice cream: bulk and packaged[61]

Similar price controls were set at the manufacturer and wholesale levels, which effectively froze the gross margin for many products. Lilly's price to wholesalers for a package of Betalin Complex was set at $1.60; the price to drugstores was set at $1.92 (a markup of 20 percent), and the price to the ultimate purchaser was $2.88 (a markup of 50 percent). Similar margins existed on items as diverse as Marlin razor blade sharpeners and Lambert's vitamins.[62] In comparison, gross margins of prescriptions ranged from 60 to 67 percent.[63] Frank A. Delgado of Washington, DC, an APhA officer before the war, served as the head of the Drugs and Fine Chemicals Unit, Chemicals and Drugs Branch of the Office of Price Administration.

Most expenses were relatively stable throughout the war period. There was little reason for the rent or utility expenses to vary much. In some cases, rents were fixed and could not change. For the most part new store construction or major remodeling did not happen; building materials and metals were in short supply. Priorities were for war production; small businesses and retailers were at the bottom of the priority list.

Several factors contributed to the exceptionally high profit margin (8.5 to 9 percent), most notable of which was a decrease in expenses (from 26 percent of sales to 22 to 23 percent) and an increase in prescription sales (from 13.2 percent in 1941 to 18.9 percent in 1945). As the drugstore went beyond the break-even point in sales (and most did in the wartime years), the fixed expenses or costs were covered. Additional sales beyond the break-even point were reduced by the cost of goods sold and variable expenses only. The remainder was net profit.[64]

MANPOWER

Manpower was in short supply. The military grew to a force of almost 12 million before the end of hostilities; there was virtually full employment of men and, in addition, 5 million women entered the workforce. The war industries were hiring at wages much higher than those offered in the retail work: if the war plant job was classified as essential, it would be easier (for those so inclined) to gain draft deferment. Pharmacists could earn more by taking jobs in production than they could in filling prescriptions. Owners had to pay higher wages for all employees or risk losing them to work in the war plants. Three factors fostered the continuing decline in the number of licensed pharmacists available for retail work:

1. The decline in graduates from the colleges of pharmacy
2. Military service—whether draft or enlistment, pharmacists were not occupationally deferred from serving
3. Competition from other employers

There were not enough pharmacists to keep the 54,500 stores open.[65] In 1942 only 72,000 pharmacists were engaged in retail work; the national average number of pharmacists per store was 1.2. Three thousand pharmacists were engaged in hospital practice.

The number of pharmacists would continue to decline as the military manpower needs increased in 1943 and 1944. According to a wage scale published in the *New Jersey Journal of Pharmacy,* the minimum wage for a registered pharmacist in 1944 was $285 per month for a forty-eight-hour workweek.[66] The compensation data for 1946 from the Elliott Report, *General Report of the Pharmaceutical Survey,* provide a more representative picture of $300 to $350 for a fifty-five to fifty-nine-hour week.[67] No matter what the salary, there was no shortage of jobs.

Although there was no national census, some states reported the number of pharmacists who were in the military. Tennessee reported that half of all male pharmacists under age thirty-five were in the service by January 1943[68] and that by February 1944, 202 pharmacists were serving.[69] By April 1943, a state board survey showed 4,530 pharmacists employed in Ohio and 320 in the Armed Forces.[70] In August 1943, 15 percent of New York pharmacists were in the military.[71] In December 1944, Utah reported that almost 9 percent (thirty-three of 376) of licensed pharmacists were in the military.[72] In October 1943 the North Carolina State Board announced that the usual November examination had been canceled: there were few candidates and they were unable to get to Chapel Hill.[73]

Drugstore owners explored a number of ways to deal with the shortage of help. In the early 1940s the typical drugstore was open 8 a.m. to 11 p.m. or midnight (approximately sixteen hours), seven days a week, or about 112 hours. The first response was a general move to decrease open hours. In some areas the owners worked together and everybody reduced the time that the stores were open. This usually resulted in opening later and closing earlier. In some areas stores took turns closing early or reducing hours on Sundays. This re-

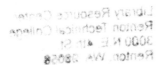

duced the workweek to an average ninety-six hours, still a much higher average than other retail stores.[74] Some owners around military camps were able to make arrangements with pharmacists in the service to do some relief work. Gregory Hartlaub, a 1942 graduate of the Cincinnati College of Pharmacy, enlisted in September 1942 and was assigned to the Station Hospital at Camp Wheeler, Georgia. He recalled helping out in a drugstore in nearby Macon, Georgia, where he worked three nights a week for several months.[75]

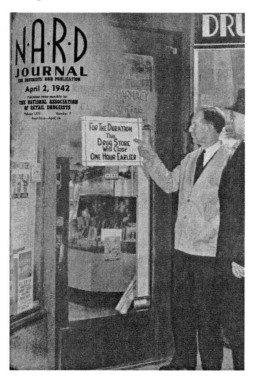

Before the war many drugstores were open sixteen hours a day, seven days a week. Manpower shortages forced many owners to decrease the number of hours a store was open. In some areas all of the stores agreed to the hours they would be open and provided a revolving list of stores that would open in the case of an emergency. (*Source: NARD Journal* [1942] 64 [April 2]: cover. Reprinted with permission. Photo courtesy of the Lloyd Library and Museum.)

Store deliveries were curtailed in most areas. While personnel was one reason, the greater reason was the rationing of gas and rubber. Nonmilitary production of cars was suspended in 1941.[76] Some stores maintained delivery services for prescriptions only, and in many areas bicycles were the vehicle of choice for the delivery boy.

Other suggestions for dealing with the shortage of pharmacists were offered. Among them was the possibility that stores with more than one pharmacist could reduce staff, thus allowing the released individual to take over the store of a man called into service. Another suggestion was to encourage owners of small stores to close or sell their business and go to work in stores with greater volume, especially in areas with a concentration of war plants.[77] Another effort called men out of retirement, even if they could only work part-time. Perhaps the most alarming suggestion for handling the manpower

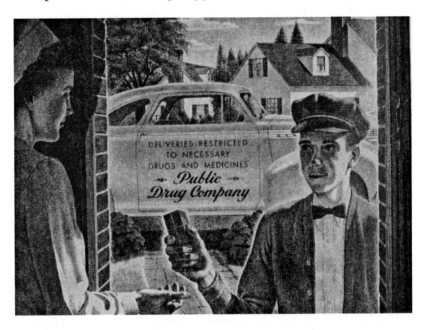

Drugstores were not eligible for extra gas rations, and delivery services using cars were virtually abandoned due to rationing of tires and gas. Some stores used other means to deliver essential medicines, but for many delivery was a service that was discontinued until the end of the war. (*Source: Pacific Drug Review* [1943] 55:24. Photo courtesy of the Lloyd Library and Museum.)

shortage came from the Tennessee director of Selective Service. He suggested that prescription centers be established in the state and noted that one center with fifteen pharmacists could serve the entire city and county of Knoxville.[78]

Many owners saw women as a possible answer to the professional manpower shortage. However, some owners refused to hire a "girl pharmacist" no matter what the manpower shortages were.[79] In the city of Waterboro, South Carolina, every store had hired one or two women to take the place of a man. Many of the women were wives of soldiers and the owners were delighted with the quality of the work, but this help would be lost when their soldier-husbands moved on to different assignments.[80] Help-wanted ads began to appear with preferences for women pharmacists because more women were graduating from pharmacy schools and they were not subject to the draft.[81] The women viewed pharmacy as an opportunity to render patriotic wartime service and to participate in a valuable professional postwar service.[82] One article summed up the issue of manpower shortages and women adroitly: "Rich indeed is the druggist today who has a large family—especially if most of them are daughters!"[83] Virginia Dolezal, a 1940 graduate of the University of Kansas, worked in her family's store in Wilson, Kansas, and at several pharmacies that had lost pharmacists until full-time replacements could be found. She also worked relief for pharmacists who went to visit sons before they were shipped overseas.[84] Anita Battista Meek graduated in 1940 from Indianapolis College of Pharmacy along with her brother. When he enlisted in the Navy, she took over running his store. She recalled that it was difficult: "We compounded lotions, creams, cough syrups, eye preparations, capsules and even suppositories. Merchandise was rationed and help was hard to find."[85]

In 1943 Sylvester Dretzka, secretary of the Wisconsin Board of Pharmacy and a national leader, posed a question of whether men would be supplanted by women in pharmacy. While he was positive toward the abilities of women, his concluding remarks focused on the verb *supplanted:*

> Few women are interested in entering the profession and of those who do enter, few devote a whole lifetime to it. And the war will probably not see any great change in this condition, al-

though an influx of women would enrich the profession. If women are to supplant men in pharmacy, it will take at least 20 to 30 years. However, the postwar period may hold some surprises in this regard.[86]

PRESCRIPTIONS

While not completely due to the war, the work in the prescription area was changing. The number of prescriptions written and filled during the war increased due to improved health awareness, fewer physicians dispensing their own remedies, and fewer drugstores. At the same time, the nature of what was being dispensed was changing. A 1942 survey showed that over 70 percent of the prescriptions dispensed did not require compounding. Most of the prescriptions that were compounded were dispensed as liquids, powders and salts, or ointments/suppositories. On average, there were three ingredients in the compounded prescriptions and almost 45 percent of all compounded prescriptions had only two.[87] A Lilly executive, Dale Ruedig, speaking at the Minnesota state association meeting in 1942, emphasized the importance of the prescription department. He noted that the average physician wrote $1,000 worth of prescriptions a year, an amount equivalent to the average purchases of twenty-five families, and encouraged owners to go after all of the prescription business they could. For perspective he noted that the prescription department represented less than 20 percent of the total store volume while producing up to 60 percent of the net profit.[88]

In 1944 two state prescription surveys were completed under the sponsorship of pharmacy schools. A statewide survey in North Carolina showed that less than 22 percent of all prescriptions were compounded; in the stores surveyed the percentage ranged from 12 percent to 38 percent.[89] An Iowa study by the Drake University College of Pharmacy defined compounding broadly to include simple solutions, mixtures, and dilutions. Just over 22 percent of the prescriptions were compounded. Over 50 percent of all prescriptions specified a brand-name product or specified the manufacturer. The study noted that the value of the pharmacist was changing from the ability to compound complicated prescriptions to the knowledge and understanding of new pharmaceuticals.[90] Both studies raised the question of curriculum adjustments to prepare students for different practice requirements than had been the case before the war.

HOSPITALS

Pharmacists in the hospital faced many of the same problems as those in the retail setting, including manpower shortages and product availability. However, there were fewer hospitals than retail pharmacies, and many of them did not have full-time pharmacists. Manpower shortages were a concern, although less publicized than those of the drugstores. The 1943 brief, "In Support of the Continued Classification of Pharmacy As an Essential Activity Under Health and Welfare Service, the Continued Deferment of Pharmacists, and a Provision for the Training of an Adequate Number of Pharmacists," reported 2,698 pharmacists working full-time in hospitals with an additional 533 working part-time, and added that this was a 16 percent increase over the previous year.[91] In May 1943 Troy Daniels of the University of California College of Pharmacy called attention to a potential source of manpower in a letter published in hospital journals. Daniels pointed out that men and women in their twenties and early thirties, graduates of the college of pharmacy, were interested in jobs outside of California. He emphasized that all of them were American-born citizens of Japanese descent.[92] In what was obviously incomplete data, NABP reported that as of December 31, 1944, 1,797 pharmacists were working in 622 hospital pharmacies.[93] The U.S. Department of Census reported 6,611 hospitals in 1944, but no data are provided on the number of those with pharmacies.[94] Although a postwar figure, the American Hospital Association noted in 1947 that only 42 percent of hospitals, 2,625 of 6,173 reporting, had hospital pharmacies.[95]

Many hospital pharmacies included a manufacturing unit to make some of their own products. This was considered by some as both a conservation mechanism and a way to reduce or control costs on ingredients. Lawrence Templeton was a pharmacist at the University of Illinois College of Pharmacy that provided pharmacy services to the University of Illinois Research and Educational Hospital. Formulas were derived that departed from prewar NF and USP standards but

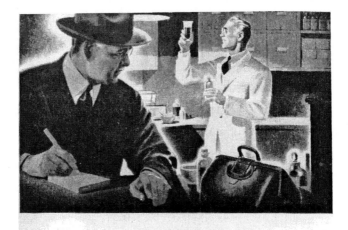

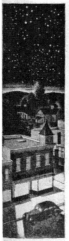

When the final chapter in the history of World War II is written ... the men and women on the home front will come in for a full share of credit. No contribution will be more glorious than that of the retail druggist, who has worked harder and longer than ever before, helping the doctor maintain that civilian health so necessary to full-time production of war materials and supplies.

Your Lilly man isn't doing as much for you as he would like. He can't get quinine for you. Some of the vitamins are scarce from time to time. Certain sulfa drugs occasionally drop from the market for a few days. Elixirs are difficult because of the shortage of glycerin. Some of the things you formerly bought in gallons are now available only in pints.

But he, like you, is doing the best he can. And you can depend most implicitly on one thing—he isn't playing any favorites. He will give you a break whenever he can. And what is more, he continues to work with your physicians in anticipation of better times to come. In war or peace your Lilly man works for you, never against you. That is the Lilly Policy. ELI LILLY AND COMPANY, Indianapolis 6, Indiana.

J. W. Ross, the senior Lilly medical service representative in Miami, Florida, joined the organization in 1923. Illness forced a short leave of absence in 1925, but since that time Mr. Ross has been on the job constantly, calling on the physicians and pharmacists of Miami, many of whom he numbers among his personal friends.

WE PAY HIM BUT HE WORKS FOR YOU   *Lilly*

NORTH WESTERN DRUGGIST   OCTOBER, 1943   29

While there were shortages of medicinal components, such as glycerin, during the war, the *United States Pharmacopoeia* and *National Formulary* devised acceptable substitutes for many items. Civilian health was important to maintain production; health supplies for civilians were a responsibility of the War Production Board Division of Chemicals, Drugs, and Health Supplies which was headed by Robert Fischelis, a pharmacist from New Jersey and the secretary of the American Pharmaceutical Association in 1945. (*Source: Northwestern Druggist* [1943] 51[October]:29. Photo courtesy of the Lloyd Library and Museum.)

were tested to assure effectiveness and meet other standards, such as rancidity for topical preparations. Examples included the substitution of bentonite magma and lime water for distilled water in the NF formula for Lotion Calamine and corn oil fortified with oleic acid for olive oil in Liniment Calamine.[96]

At least some hospitals had implemented a formulary system, seemingly aimed at encouraging the use of standard USP items for simplification of stock and potential cost savings. Fischelis and Mordell noted that it was important to have a strong pharmacy committee and that the standards of both the American College of Surgeons and the American Hospital Association's Committee on Pharmacy supported such committees. The authors also provided an overview of some of the War Production Board's orders that had an impact on hospitals. These included the use of agar for bacteriological media, nutgalls and tannic acid for burns, and vitamin A, as well as tin tubes and quinine.[97] Robert Fuqua, chief pharmacist of the Johns Hopkins Hospital in Baltimore, continued the theme of shortages and conservation later in the year. Imports of such products as castor beans, coconut oil, Chinese cinnamon, and menthol were still interrupted by the war, but adequate substitutes could be developed. However, he noted that one of the most significant problems was the shortage of alcohol and the continuing need to devise substitutes. Hospitals used vast quantities of 75 percent alcohol, much of it for nightly backrubs, and found that suggested 35 percent concentrations were not nearly as effective. The alternative developed was to substitute a 60 percent USP alcohol with a trace of zinc phenolsulfonate for astringency, 2 percent glycerin as a skin lubricant, 3 percent acetone to increase absorption, and a trace of aromatic oil for scent. This formulation saved hospitals over 100 gallons of alcohol per month.[98]

Chapter 6

Pharmacy Corps

On July 12, 1943, Franklin Delano Roosevelt signed the Durham-Reynolds Bill as Public Law 130 establishing the Pharmacy Corps in the U.S. Army. This simple act brought an official closure to a long-standing struggle for professional recognition between organized pharmacy and the Army. While the signing was a historic moment, the true impact was the acceptance of pharmacy as a profession—a victory that long outlived the Pharmacy Corps.

The drive to establish the corps began at the 1894 annual APhA meeting in Asheville, North Carolina.[1] Progress in the intervening forty-nine years was intermittent, moving forward in spurts during military conflicts and then lying fallow during times of peace. Little did Atlanta pharmacist George F. Payne realize what his original resolution at the 1894 APhA meeting would entail before the Army recognized pharmacy as a profession.

THE BEGINNING

A commissioned pharmacy service existed in the U.S. Army until it was eliminated for financial reasons in 1818. Andrew Craigie, an iconic figure in pharmacy history, was the apothecary general in the Revolutionary War. The duty of the pharmacist was "to receive, prepare and deliver medicines and other articles of his department to the hospitals and army."[2] Less well known, James Cutbush served as one of the apothecary generals during the War of 1812. At the conclusion of the war, funds were restricted and the military was severely reduced in size. Cutbush became the professor of chemistry at West Point and the apothecary general's position disappeared from the Army table of organization. The role of the pharmacist in the Civil

War was much less defined compared to earlier conflicts. There was no apothecary general and no pharmacists were commissioned to serve as pharmacists; those who served as pharmacists were enlisted hospital stewards. Civilian contractors and military purveyors carried out the procurement functions. Thus in a period of less than 100 years the Army had demoted the rank and role of the apothecary from one deemed important enough for a commission to that of an artisan or a common soldier.

At the 1894 APhA annual meeting, George F. Payne of Atlanta, Georgia, introduced a resolution to seek recognition of pharmacy in the U.S. Army and Navy. APhA president Edgar L. Patch appointed the Special Committee on the Status of Pharmacists in the Army and Navy of the United States with Payne as chair. Each state, the Indian Territory, and the District of Columbia had a representative on the committee, two of whom were women (Mary O. Miner of Kansas and Nellie C. Hall of South Dakota).[3]

By the 1895 APhA meeting the committee had prepared draft legislation based on its survey of the status of pharmacists in the military organizations of Europe and Japan.* The committee bills for the Army, Navy, and Marine Hospital Service were introduced in the 54th Congress by Senator A. O. Bacon and Representative Charles F. Crisp. Rather than seek commissions, the bills provided for recognition in position and pay for pharmacists as well as the requirement that those assigned to pharmaceutical duties be graduates in pharmacy. However, all of the services adamantly opposed the legislation, and Congress did not pass any of the bills.[4] Army Surgeon General Sternberg's opposition was the beginning of a struggle that would last through the terms of ten different surgeons general.

The committee did gain some advances for pharmacists in the Navy and Marine Hospital Service, the precursor of the Public Health Service. In response to invitations to send representatives, both the Navy and the Public Health and Marine Hospital Service sent official delegations to the 1903 annual meeting of the American Pharmaceutical Association. There was also a delegation from Harvey Wiley's National Bureau of Control of Medicines and Foods of the Depart-

---

*In the U.S. Navy apothecaries were enlisted men and were outranked by boatswains, gunners, carpenters, and sail makers, all of whom were warrant officers. APhA (1895). *Proceedings of the APhA,* 43:96.

ment of Agriculture. The Army Surgeon General O'Reilly refused to send representatives stating that the "position of pharmacist or apothecary does not exist in the Army."[5]

Beginning in 1912 the APhA committee shifted its efforts to respond to changes in the Army. The pay scales and authorized strength of the service had changed, putting the enlisted men in the Hospital Corps at a disadvantage. For example, privates caring for the sick were paid eighteen dollars per month while farriers who worked under veterinarians caring for sick mules and horses were paid twenty-one dollars per month. In the Navy, the first class hospital apprentice, a rank comparable to the private first class in the Army, earned thirty-three dollars per month.[6] Senator Augustus Bacon and Representative Hughes introduced legislation in the 62nd Congress to change the name of the Hospital Corps to Medical Corps and to establish pay parity. Organized pharmacy lent support to the bill in the belief that a rising tide lifts all ships and that the better pay and increased opportunity for promotion in the noncommissioned ranks would result in better men, including pharmacists, entering and staying in the service. The Bacon-Hughes legislation was drafted with the support of the surgeon general but was opposed by the secretary of war. In reviewing the 1914 effort, W. B. Day, a Chicago pharmacist and APhA president in 1911-1912, reported that the committee favored asking for commissions for pharmacists. The basis for the request included a familiar refrain: "it would be a recognition of the professional status of pharmacists."[7]

WORLD WAR I PERIOD

At the 1915 annual meeting of the APhA in San Francisco, Caswell Mayo gave a high priority to the issue of pharmacists in the military in his presidential address. He acknowledged the success of the Committee on the Status of Pharmacists in the Government Service in improving the lot of pharmacists in the Navy and Public Health Service but noted that there was no similar success in the Army. He argued that success might have been more evident if effort had been placed on the creation of a new medical service rather than improving the lot of individuals. Consequently, he recommended that the Committee on the Status of Pharmacists in the Government Service be instructed to draft and seek passage by Congress of a bill providing for the creation of a corps of highly educated expert pharmacists, whose duty shall be to direct the medical supply service of the United States Army, and to continue their efforts toward the betterment of the status of the men now in the service.[8]

Samuel Hilton, the new chair of the Committee on the Status of Pharmacists in the Government Service, noted that Congress was busy with issues relating to the European conflict. He also assessed that the reintroduction of the Hughes Bill (Bacon had died in 1914) would continue to face strong opposition from the secretary of war and recommended that APhA work with the surgeon general to address opposition.[9]

Hilton's strategy worked; at the 1916 annual meeting he reported that Army Surgeon General Gorgas was able to gain enough support to secure passage of the Hughes Bill. The results were the reorganization of the Hospital Corps into the Medical Department of the Army. New noncommissioned ranks were established and pay scales increased; however, a separate pharmacy corps was not established, nor were pharmacists commissioned. Hilton also reported on a positive interaction with the Secretary of the Navy Josephus Daniels,* noting that Daniels was pleasant to deal with and had been connected with the drug trade in his youth.[10]

On April 2, 1917, Woodrow Wilson called for a declaration of war against Germany; the draft quickly brought large numbers of men into uniform. To gain support of a pharmacy corps from physicians, Joseph W. England of the Philadelphia College of Pharmacy wrote a letter to the editor of the *Journal of the American Medical Association*. He pointed out that medicine had not shirked its military duties and called for support of the establishment of a pharmacy corps and "proper professional recognition so that it may have the opportunity to do its fullest and best work for the sick and wounded."[11] A cover-

---

*Josephus Daniels was from North Carolina. During his youth he worked in several odd jobs, including clerking in a drugstore. He became a successful newspaper publisher. Wilson appointed him secretary of the Navy, and he served from 1913 to 1921. State Library of North Carolina, North Carolina Encyclopedia, <http://statelibrary.dcr.stte.nc.us/nc/ncbiz/daniels.htm>.

ing editorial pointed out that "victory in war goes to the nation that most effectively conserves the health of its fighting men" and supported pharmacy's cause first, because it is only just and, second, because the medical corps will be made more effective.[12] APhA President Frederick Wulling wrote to Newton Baker, the secretary of war, restating pharmacy's desire for a commissioned corps responsible for the medical supply service of the Army. Baker replied pleasantly enough but provided a copy of a letter from Surgeon General Gorgas expressing his satisfaction with the status quo and opposition to commissioning pharmacists. Samuel Hilton, the chair of the APhA Committee of the Status of Pharmacists in the Government Service, enlisted the aid of Dr. W. J. Mayo (one of the Mayo brothers of Minneapolis, who served as an advisor to Gorgas) in setting a meeting with the surgeon general. Hilton reported that the meeting was short and marked by considerable antagonism toward the establishment of a separate corps.[13]

There was dissatisfaction with the progress that was being made in gaining a separate pharmacy corps. During the 1917 APhA meeting, its past president, George Beringer, discussed the formation of the National Pharmaceutical Service Association. Representatives of four organizations—the Philadelphia Branch of the American Pharmaceutical Association, the Philadelphia Association of Retail Druggists, the Philadelphia Drug Exchange, and the Philadelphia College of Pharmacy—agreed that the most important goal was to establish a pharmacy corps and, with it, a reserve component. This group developed a bill that was presented by Representative George Edmonds, a pharmacist and graduate of the Philadelphia College of Pharmacy. Beringer asked the APhA to support the Edmonds legislation.[14]

Also at the 1917 APhA meeting, Francis Edward Stewart, a Philadelphia physician and pharmacist, summarized the Edmonds Bill as well as the current activities by a number of pharmacy groups at the Section on Education and Legislation. The Edmonds Bill, HR 5531, set the stage for all of the interests of organized pharmacy in its full title, "To Increase the Efficiency of the Medical Department of the United States Army, to Provide a Pharmaceutical Corps in that department, and to Improve the Status and Efficiency of the Pharmacists in the Army." Stewart's paper provided an important insight to the military's opposition to the establishment of the separate pharmacy corps. He had heard from military leaders the concern that the creation of such a corps would legitimatize the "nostrum business." Stewart noted that it was common practice for physicians to prescribe and pharmacists to sell proprietary products, those used for "domestic" treatment and used the example of cough remedies. The role of the pharmacist, Stewart added, "was to be the expert in the knowledge of drugs and their uses, not an expert in the knowledge of diseases and their treatment." Stewart believed that the Edmonds Bill, while dealing with military pharmacy, would also have a positive influence on civilian practice.

> We believe that it would give the prestige and influence to the practitioners of true pharmacy in the United States. We believe that it would excite interest in pharmaceutical education and thus promote the welfare of our educational institutions. We believe that it would aid in restoring the confidence of the medical profession and the public generally in drugs as remedial agents, and thus materially promote the public health.[15]

Army Surgeon General Gorgas continued his opposition, apparently without ever providing his basis for it beyond stating that pharmacists were not necessary and that he preferred the status quo. In the absence of justification there had to be speculation about his position. Joseph England questioned whether it was because he was

> preeminently a sanitarian and not a therapeutist, and is more sympathetic to preventive medicine (of which sanitation is a branch) than to curative medicine (of which therapeutics and pharmacy are branches), as his establishment of a Sanitary Corps in the Army, while opposing the establishment of a Pharmaceutical [sic] Corps, might imply?[16]

In preparation for congressional hearings on the Edmonds Bill, the APhA Committee of the Status of Pharmacists in the Government Service sent a survey to each state board of pharmacy requesting information on how pharmacy was being practiced in the Army installations in their jurisdictions. Twenty-six replies reported

> the dispensing of medicines was often done by others than graduate pharmacists and sometimes those who had been bartend-

ers, salesmen, bookkeepers and others, without any knowledge of drugs, were in charge of dispensaries, while pharmacists under them as privates could do no dispensing except under the direction of such non-commissioned officers.[17]

The committee's annual report provided further anecdotal information on the Army establishment's opposition to the formation of the Pharmacy Corps:

Close contact with men of authority in the medical departments usually elicits the information that the pharmacists are not wanted, they know too much, that they want men without pharmaceutical training so that they can train them as they desire. The younger men in the medical service want the pharmacists, but they have not the power to overcome the opposition.[18]

In supplemental remarks to the 1918 annual report, Samuel Hilton introduced a new element to the debate for the establishment of the Corps—a statement covering universal commissioning and educational credentials. Hilton remarked on a presentation from earlier in the meeting that had suggested the commercial interests in pharmacy exceeded the educational and professional interests and that it was, in part, this imbalance which created a barrier to full recognition by the Army.[19] Hilton explained that the committee was not seeking a commission for every corner druggist but a corps made up of trained pharmacists—those "qualified in pharmacy by education and training, men who are competent to render pharmaceutical service."[20]

The House Committee on Military Affairs held hearings on HR 5531 on March 19, 1918. Frederick Wulling, dean of the University of Minnesota College of Pharmacy and president of APhA, provided the opening comments and introduced those who would testify for pharmacy. There was no testimony by anyone in the military, and the presence of no representative of the surgeon general's office was recorded. The only insight into the surgeon general's position was a copy of a memorandum circulated at the direction of the surgeon general that was included as Exhibit VIII in Wulling's testimony:

It is felt that the needs of the soldiers can be provided for satisfactorily under the present organization; that the department

will be severely taxed to provide, under the present form of organization, the essentials of medical care for our rapidly increasing Army; and that any change in the form of organization
at the present time, except such as are found necessary and are
requested by the Surgeon General, would not only delay these
essential provisions for the medical care of our soldiers but
might prevent the inauguration of a number of new and important measures planned for their benefit.[21]

The memorandum concluded that the proposed legislation is nothing
more than self-interest that should not be addressed in the current period of war. The Edmonds Bill, never sent to the floor for a vote, died
at the end of the 65th Congress.

BETWEEN THE WARS

The end of World War I brought a change in pharmacy's efforts for
military recognition. Hilton's report at the 1919 APhA meeting noted
that Gorgas's term as surgeon general was up and a new man,
Merritte W. Ireland, was appointed. Hilton's strategy, put forward in
his conclusions, was that the only way to gain recognition for pharmacy in the Army was to work with the new surgeon general.

The committee report also included information on legislation introduced by Congressman George Darrow, HR 4760, "To Increase
the Efficiency of the Medical Department of the United States Navy
and Improve the Status and Efficiency of the Hospital Corps of the
U.S. Navy." Commenting that Surgeon General of the Navy Braisted
supported the legislation, Hilton urged APhA to provide its full support since the bill provided for the establishment of a commissioned
pharmacy corps in the Navy. This concluded Hilton's involvement
with the Committee on the Status of Pharmacists in the Government
Service; E. Fullerton Cook was appointed the new chair.[22]

The 1920 committee report stated that meetings had been held
with both the Navy (Josephus Daniels and Admiral Braisted) and the
Army (General Ireland) but concluded that pharmacy had not gained
concessions from either branch. Ireland stated that educated pharmacists had made a mark for themselves and the profession during the
war and he hoped that the better ones would stay in the Army and

help organize the administrative corps. Criteria for a commission in the reserve of the Medical Administrative Corps were a high school diploma and special training, including pharmacy.[23] Late in 1920 the efforts with the Navy would gain new support with the appointment of Edward Rhodes Stitt as the surgeon general. Stitt was a pharmacist, having graduated from the Philadelphia College of Pharmacy in 1887. E. Fullerton Cook, the chair of the Committee on the Status of Pharmacists in the Government Service, graduated from PCP in 1900.

In 1921 and 1922 Cook wrote to both Ireland and Stitt seeking information on the current status of pharmacists in the respective services. Ireland responded that there were fifteen commissioned officers in the medical department who were pharmacists and thirty-seven pharmacists in the Medical Administrative Officers Corps Reserve. However, they were in management positions rather than practicing pharmacy. Ireland also responded that he was in favor of more slots for trained pharmacists in administrative positions. Stitt's reply, while cordial, spoke to the difficulty in gaining commissions for those practicing pharmacy. The conclusions that Cook drew in his APhA report both echoed and foretold the continuing effort to gain commissions and a separate corps. Qualified pharmacists were being commissioned, but not as pharmacists. However, in order to gain a commission the individual had to be "well trained professionally and have other qualifications essential for success as an officer."[24] In August of 1922, Ireland invited applications for the Medical Administrative Reserve by qualified pharmacists who were recommended by the American Pharmaceutical Association or the dean of a college of pharmacy.[25] By 1923 eighty-nine pharmacists held commissions in the Medical Administrative Corps and an additional twenty-five were in the Sanitary Corps.[26] In 1924 several bills circulated for establishing pharmacist commissions in the Navy but were not introduced; graduation from a recognized college of pharmacy would be one of the requirements.[27]

Contention over the absence of success in the search for military recognition erupted again during the 1928 annual APhA meeting. Cook made the usual report of lack of progress with both the Army and the Navy. The Navy was not (and had never been) the primary objective because it was the smaller of the military branches. The target of displeasure was the Army. The surgeon general was backing legislation for the creation of the Medical Service Corps, which would incorporate the current Medical Administrative Corps, the Sanitary Corps, and an enlisted complement from the medical and dental sections. While pharmacists could be commissioned, there would be no separate, commissioned pharmacy section. In response to the Army's intransigence a draft bill was prepared for the creation of the separate Pharmacy Corps. This draft was likely influenced or developed by pharmacists serving at Walter Reed Army Hospital since it grandfathered those without a four-year college education:

> To commission about twenty-two registered pharmacists now in the military service and who have actually been engaged in strictly pharmaceutical duties of sufficient importance within the military service and for a long enough period to justify their claim to such recognition despite their probable lack of 4-years' college of pharmacy work, and also provides for the commissioning at a later date of thirty-three or more, better trained pharmacists than the army now has in its service, to complete the initial allowance of the Corps; and further provides that all future vacancies occurring in the Corps shall be filled by such 4-year college of pharmacy graduates.[28]

A. G. DuMez, chair of the Special Committee to Consider the Proposed Bill for the Establishment of a Pharmacy Corps in the U.S. Army, recommended support of the proposed bill. An interchange between DuMez and Cook exposed the difference in approach that existed between the regular committee and the special committee. Cook admitted to his opposition to establish a separate pharmacy corps, arguing for cooperation with the surgeon general and the support of his planned reorganization that would integrate pharmacy into the new corps. DuMez's response was that cooperation had resulted in little advance over the thirty years of effort. The resolution of the special committee was passed.

The proposed bill tacitly recognized that the different levels of education were an issue—not only in the military but for pharmacy. The veiled comments about qualifications and education boiled to the surface with the recognition of differences between the older men and the four-year graduates. Also at issue was the basic question about what the proper strategy would be in relation to the surgeon general's office—confrontation or cooperation. What DuMez seemed to have forgotten, if he ever knew, was that the confrontation between pharmacy and the Army during Gorgas's term as surgeon general was far less productive in gaining pay and status for the pharmacist than the approach used during Cook's tenure which was based on developing an understanding with the Army.

Representative Clyde Kelly of Pennsylvania introduced a bill to create a pharmacy corps in the medical department of the U.S. Army. A companion bill was introduced in the Senate by Royal Copeland of New York. Hearings on HR 16278 were held before the House Committee on Military Affairs on February 20, 1929. As was the case in the 1918 hearings on the Edmonds Bill, no representatives of the surgeon general's office testified. Surgeon General Ireland was not receptive to a request for a meeting; instead his position was set out in a letter to A. L. I. Winnie, the new chair of the APhA Committee on Pharmacy Corps in the U.S. Army. Ireland stated there was an agreement with E. Fullerton Cook and the American Pharmaceutical Association that a mutually satisfactory compromise would be reached if pharmacists were allowed to be commissioned in the Medical Administrative Corps. Ireland objected to the establishment of too many constituent corps and stated that he would be opposed to the creation of any pharmacy corps as long as he was surgeon general. Winnie responded to Ireland including a statement from Cook that there never was such an agreement and that he had never been in a position to bind the APhA to such an agreement.

During the hearings, pharmacy took the opportunity to explain how the establishment of such a corps would help the surgeon general. In his testimony, Hilton, who had been chair of the APhA committee from 1915 to 1919 and was both a pharmacist and a physician, discussed several prescriptions for soldiers that had been written by a military physician and caught in error by an observant pharmacist. One prescription called for 1,000 grams of morphine or 2.2 pounds— an equivalent to a medicinal dose of morphine for 60,000 people. The second prescription was for 5,000 grams of 10 percent boric acid ointment—enough to use in the eyes of every man, woman, and child in both Washington, DC, and New York City. The final example was for 200 grams of chloral hydrate—over 200 doses of the sedative.[29] There was no action on the bill.

During the 1929 annual APhA meeting A. L. I. Winnie suggested a future course of action calling for public relations with patriotic and fraternal organizations and sustained political action with members of congress who had seats on various military committees. James H. Beal moved for acceptance of the committee report and added that "this was one time that the representatives of pharmacy had the courage to say what they believed . . . the committees representing pharmacy had always permitted themselves to be side-tracked and put off with promises."[30]

The official response of the surgeon general's office was published in the November 1929 issue of the *Army and Navy Register* under the title "Irregular Legislative Schemes." The article dismissed the Kelly Bill as being of little consequence. The article stated that the surgeon general did not know where the bill to establish a pharmacy corps originated but assumed that it was aided and abetted by the association of pharmacists. The author dismissed information on dangerous prescribing by Army medical officers as making no impression on the House Committee. In a *Journal of the American Pharmaceutical Association (JAPhA)* editorial, Robert Swain, the NABP president, replied caustically that there was no doubt who put forward the Kelly Bill; the Winnie correspondence proved that. Swain concluded his editorial with the charge that the military provided less protection for human life than was available on the civilian side—an argument that would become more compelling as the peace-time Army of less than 1 million men gave way to the wartime military of 12 million.

> It is obvious that life, health and happiness are not given the same high value in military circles that is accorded these priceless possessions where a human being is still a human being irrespective of his position in the social cosmos.[31]

In 1929 Jonathan Wainwright of New York, a member of the House Committee on Military Affairs, introduced a bill to change the organization of the Medical Corps with the full support of the surgeon general and the secretary of war. His legislation made no provision for a separate, commissioned Pharmacy Corps; instead, the chief thrust of the legislation was the replacement of the Medical Administrative Corps with the Medical Auxiliary Corps. No hearings were held on this legislation.

During the 1930 APhA meeting the Committee on the Pharmacy Corps in the U.S. Army reported that bills to create a pharmacy corps had been reintroduced in both Houses with several strategic moves. Brazilla Reece of Tennessee, a member of the powerful Military Affairs Committee, put forward the House bill in place of Clyde Kelly. Senator Copeland, a physician, reintroduced his bill with the expectation that his expertise on medical matters would gain support. Both the surgeon general and the secretary of war continued their opposition. Pharmacy's strategy was to continue to increase the flow of information to Congress.[32]

Inaccurate dispensing caused a public relations nightmare for the Army. In April two children of two enlisted men died as a result of an error in dispensing. The physician wrote for atropine sulfate hypodermic tablets, dissolved and given in drops. Not having the hypodermic tablets, and understanding neither the strength nor the dosage, powdered atropine sulfate was weighed and used; the dispenser was an Army corporal who had no pharmacy training but was responsible for dispensing at Fort Leavenworth. Court martial proceedings were held; the corporal was acquitted and returned to his dispensing duties.[33] In a *JAPhA* editorial Swain quoted the *El Dorado Times:* "Surely the lives of soldiers and their dependents are entitled to be safeguarded against ignorance and inexperience. The Army certainly needs the services of pharmacists who know their business."[34]

The year 1931 brought a number of changes in the continuing struggle between pharmacy and the Army. Merritte W. Ireland's term as surgeon general was concluding; Robert Patterson's was beginning. During the year the APhA Committee met with each of the surgeon generals at their invitation; each indicated that pharmacy in the military must be changed and improved. The sticking point became whether this could be better accomplished with the Wainwright Bill or the Reese-Copeland Bill. The Army was not willing to establish a separate pharmacy corps but would recommend the establishment of a separate pharmacy section in the Medical Auxiliary Corps. Swain pointed out that organized pharmacy's objective was "adequate and dependable pharmaceutical service," the name was of secondary importance, and pharmacy was more likely to achieve its ends by working with the surgeon general.[35]

The relationship between Surgeon General Patterson and pharmacy was based on the mutual agreement that the status of pharmaceutical services must be improved; the question was how to achieve it. Patterson remained adamantly opposed to the formation of a separate corps but was willing to commit to a separate division in the planned Auxiliary Corps. This agreement was not to be consummated in the passage of new legislation as the country entered the Great Depression in 1932 and plans to reorganize the Army were put on hold.

Swain's 1934 committee report at APhA once again recapitulated Surgeon General Patterson's position on the improvement of pharmaceutical services and the opposition to a separate pharmacy corps. However, other forces were at work in pharmacy. Swain noted that:

> Your Committee has received serious objections from several prominent pharmacists to the scheme of the Surgeon General, whereby pharmacists would be commissioned in the proposed Medical Auxiliary Corps, because in their opinion pharmacy would always be subordinated where there was any conflict of interest, and that we would never have the authority or the freedom necessary to develop the highest type of pharmaceutical service. They feel, too, that our identity would be lost and medicine would reap the credit that justly belonged to pharmacy.[36]

THE KENDIG ERA

H. Evert Kendig was appointed the chair of the Committee on Pharmacy Corps in the United States Army at the 1934 APhA annual meeting. In early 1935 a meeting was arranged with representatives of the APhA, AACP, and NABP and Surgeon General Patterson. Although the meeting was cordial, the surgeon general was candid about his plans for improving pharmaceutical services and his continued opposition to the creation of the separate Pharmacy Corps. Patterson wanted to create a new Auxiliary Corps which would include four-year pharmacy graduates. While this corps would be relatively small there would also be a reserve force that could be activated in the time of emergency. In a follow-up letter, Patterson cited a survey of the Army hospitals and noted that it would not be feasible to have highly trained and commissioned pharmacists devoted to compounding in the smaller post hospitals since little compounding was done in military institutions. The Army purchased most medicines in finished dose forms and the official supply table did not include many of the items available in the civilian pharmacy. Those pharmacists who were commissioned would have responsibility for pharmaceutical services as well as other duties expected of an officer.[37] One of the points emphasized in this meeting was that graduation from a four-year college program was the requirement for a commission. This was especially significant since the four-year mandatory course for a bachelor of science degree in pharmacy schools did not come into effect until the 1932 entering freshman class.[38] (The first college of pharmacy to institute a mandatory four-year BS was Ohio State University with the entering freshman class in 1925.)

In 1935 Charles R. Reynolds was named to succeed Robert Patterson as the Army's surgeon general. Reynolds agreed with his predecessors' efforts to establish a Medical Auxiliary Corps and use commissioned pharmacists in it. He also affirmed his opposition to the establishment of a separate pharmacy corps. At the 1935 APhA meeting the surgeon general's position was reported and Kendig's committee recommended the following:

1. That the Committee be continued and that it be instructed to continue its efforts to effect improvement in the pharmaceutical service in the Army, and to obtain therein for pharmacy the recognition and status to which it is entitled by virtue of its traditions and the useful service which it is prepared by education and training to render.
2. That the Committee be instructed to cooperate with the Surgeon General in obtaining the passage of legislation which will bring about the substance of recommendation number 1. If the objective as stated in recommendation number 1 cannot be obtained by this procedure, we recommend:
3. That the committee be instructed to obtain the desired improvement in the pharmaceutical service and its concomitant recognition in the Army by direct appeal to Congress.[39]

In 1936 Senator Morris Sheppard introduced SR 4380 restricting commissions in the Medical Administrative Corps to pharmacists. Perhaps Reynolds saw this as an effort of pharmacy to gain a back door to a separate corps and his spirit of cooperation with the APhA committee changed.[40] There was no indication in the 1935 or 1936 annual reports that the APhA committee solicited Sheppard's bill, although it clearly met the objectives of putting pharmaceutical services in the hands of pharmacists. Hearings were held in May of 1936, the legislation was passed in June, and it was signed into law as Public Law 781. The Army held exams in December; of the sixty-four pharmacists qualified to sit for the exams, two passed. Glenn K. Smith and Howard Nelson were commissioned as second lieutenants in the Medical Administrative Corps (MAC) and were assigned to general hospitals in San Francisco and Denver.[41]

In the 1940 report of the Committee on the Status of Pharmacists in the Government Service, Kendig referred to the 1936 legislation granting officer status to pharmacists as "our bill." Four separate exams had been held for commissions in the MAC, and all sixteen vacancies were filled; two remained on the eligible list. Kendig commented that there was some pressure in pharmacy circles to obtain additional appointments quickly. But this would not be the strategy since influential friends (unnamed) were providing advice on when and how to meet pharmacy's objectives.[42]

In his presidential address at the 1941 APhA annual meeting in Detroit, President Charles H. Evans included a clarion call "to enlist the support of an organized pharmacy in demanding a separate Pharmacy Corps. *NOW.* This is the opportune time. We should not delay." [43] A war was raging in Europe and Asia; a universal draft that included pharmacists and pharmacy students was operating in the United States; and the size of the American military was rapidly increasing. In response, the convention passed two resolutions. The first (Resolution 10) instructed the Committee on the Status of Pharmacists in the Government Service to promote the establishment of a separate pharmacy corps by congressional action. The second (Resolution 22) established public health and safety as the basis for the establishment of the separate corps:

Whereas, in the interest of public safety and welfare the distribution, compounding and dispensing of medicines is now legally restricted to persons who have demonstrated their competency through examination and have been licensed by the Board of Pharmacy of the state in which they practice, and

Whereas, it is no less necessary that the personnel of the military, naval, and other governmental services be afforded the same protection in the matter of preparing and distributing medication as is accorded them in civil life,

Be it Resolved, that the assignment of duties connected with the compounding and dispensing of drugs and medicines in the armed forces be restricted to persons duly licensed to practice pharmacy, and

Be it Further Resolved, that copies of this resolution be transmitted by the American Pharmaceutical Association to the Surgeon General of the United States Army, the members of the Military Affairs Committee of the Senate and to the members of the Military Affairs Committee of the House of Representatives.[44]

The lines were being drawn for the final struggle for professional recognition of pharmacy between the Army and organized pharmacy.

In 1942 a new committee was formed to coordinate the efforts of four pharmacy groups—the American Pharmaceutical Association (APhA), the National Association of Boards of Pharmacy (NABP), the American Association of Colleges of Pharmacy (AACP), and the National Association of Retail Druggists (NARD). E. F. Kelley represented the APhA. Kendig, chair of both the APhA and AACP Committees on the Status of the Pharmacists in Government Service, represented both bodies. Robert Swain, the NABP representative, had served earlier as the chair of the APhA Committee on the Status of Pharmacists in the Government Service. Roland Jones represented NARD.

The committee's first task, to develop a bill and find a sponsor in Congress, was not especially formidable. The starting point for the draft legislation was the Sheppard Bill, which required that the officers of the Medical Administrative Corps be pharmacists. Congressman Carl Durham from Chapel Hill, North Carolina, a member of the

House Military Affairs Committee, was the perfect choice. He had served as a Navy pharmacist mate during WWI and had graduated from the University of North Carolina's School of Pharmacy in 1918. The draft legislation was provided to then Surgeon General James C. Magee in an attempt to gain his support for the creation of the Pharmacy Corps. Magee declined to support pharmacy's bill but did support the May Bill to raise the maximum rank in the Medical Administrative Corps from captain to colonel. The Pharmacy committee adopted the strategy of withholding their legislation until the May bill was passed and the higher ranks assured.

Carl Durham introduced HR 7432, "To Create a Pharmacy Corps in the United States Army" on July 23, 1942. Robert Reynolds of North Carolina, the chair of the Senate's Committee on Military Affairs, introduced a companion bill, SR 2690, a week later. The legislation covered only the regular Army; the activated reserve corps and those in the service for the period of the wartime emergency were excluded.

Durham's bill had only four provisions. The first provision was to change the name of the current Medical Administrative Corps to the Pharmacy Corps; all of the current serving officers were pharmacists. The second provision was to increase the authorized strength from sixteen pharmacists to seventy-two. The third provision was to provide a promotion ladder comparable to the rest of the Army's Medical Department. The fourth provision was to create a reserve corps so that the regular Army could be expanded quickly in the state of emergency. The objective of the legislation was to centralize the purchase, shipment, storage, and standardization of medical supplies under those best equipped by education and training to perform the duties, i.e., pharmacists. From the very beginning there was an understanding, at least within pharmacy leadership, that not every pharmacist in the Army would be commissioned.[45]

The House Committee on Military Affairs held hearings on Durham's HR 7432 on November 19, 1942, at the end of the second session of the 77th Congress. General Larry McAfee, the assistant to the surgeon general, was the first to be heard. McAfee stated that the proposed legislation did not have the support of the military and added that "the safeguarding of and compounding of prescriptions, is now provided in our hospitals and our field installations, and that the technical service rendered by registered pharmacists does not demand or merit a commission."[46] The House committee explored a number of issues during the general's testimony, but most of the attention focused on the fairness of the Army's treatment of educated professionals as well as the tasks of military pharmacists. McAfee averred that the role of the pharmacist was technical, similar to that of an X-ray technician, simply responding to a physician's order. He stated that most of the medicines used were already in final dose forms and properly labeled so that any "intelligent boy can read the label. And he knows the dangerous ones."[47] Pennsylvania Congressman Ivor Fenton, who was also a physician and a veteran of the Medical Corps in WWI, disagreed with the surgeon general's position. He testified to the importance to the physician of the pharmacist's knowledge of drugs, stating the proper use of the pharmacist allowed the physician to pay full attention to medical care. He also argued that the role of the pharmacist was not analogous to that of the X-ray technician. The pharmacist had a responsibility that could result in the death of men; the X-ray technician was responsible only for taking pictures and maintaining the machine.[48]

The first hearings concluded with General McAfee's testimony; time had run out in the legislative session. Durham reintroduced his bill at the beginning of the 78th Congress and the hearings on the newly numbered bill (HR 997) began on March 2, 1943. It was finally pharmacy's opportunity to convince the Committee on Military Affairs that the establishment of the Pharmacy Corps was the right thing to do.

Pharmacy had gathered the public opinion and political action that had first been recommended in 1929 and was prepared to use it. Twelve individuals testified, among them Governor Blood of New Hampshire, who was a physician; the executive director of the American Legion; and a number of congressmen who reported their constituents' support of pharmacists.

Pharmacy leaders also testified. Kendig, Swain, Newton, Kelly, and Jones each took the podium along with Arthur Einbeck, a major in the inactive reserve of the Sanitary Corps and a New Jersey pharmacy leader. Other pharmacists were in the room, and from time to time a question from a member of the House committee was referred to the audience for an immediate answer. The pharmacy speakers repeatedly emphasized that the level of safety the pharmacist provided in civil life was absent in the Army, and the profession of pharmacy frequently required life and death judgments.

H. Evert Kendig took the lead in testifying for pharmacy. He pointed out that the struggle to gain recognition for pharmacy was not new. He reviewed the opposition of the Army to the creation of a separate commissioned corps, but his major thrust was that soldiers were not accorded the same protection with their medicines that civilians were. He attacked a statement that the military could not afford a pharmacist officer in a full-time dispensing function stating that the military's position was to provide an inferior service that affected the health and welfare of the individuals in the service. He concluded that their mothers and fathers would not approve of this policy. In response to the military use of ninety-day trainees as pharmacists, he pointed out that

> 26% of the men who will be rendering pharmaceutical service to our sons and daughters in the Army will have a smattering of training which, if used for the same purpose in civilian life, in any state in the Union and the District of Columbia, would promptly subject them to the penalties of the law.[49]

He continued the theme of safety with comments that pharmacists were placed under the direction of these ninety-day trainees, a practice denied by the Army. Kendig simply stated that such reports were on file with the deans of colleges in the states represented by the House committee members. Then he turned his attention to the allegation that the Army used mostly finished dose forms bearing instructions that any "intelligent boy" could read.

> I submit without fear of contradiction that even an intelligent boy cannot read those labels. Reading implies understanding. The names would be meaningless to him—just so many letters. The implication was that no pharmaceutical education is required for intelligent dispensing[50]

Kendig used an official press release from the Army to address the issue of finished dose forms:

The pharmacy fills over 18,000 prescriptions a month for major and minor illnesses—despite the fact that this post has one of the best health records in the entire country. That amount of prescriptions calls for 425 gallons of liquids, 120 pounds of ointments and 15,000 capsules.[51]

Robert Swain, a pharmacist-lawyer, presented the National Association of Boards of Pharmacy testimony to the House committee. His prepared comments recounted the fact that both pharmacists and pharmacies had to be licensed to practice in every state. During the questions Swain pointed out that commissions were of secondary importance in the establishment of the Pharmacy Corps since only seventy-two men could be commissioned. The primary goal was to make pharmaceutical service in the military safe, a condition that it did not currently enjoy.

> We have every reason to believe that there are men engaged in the United States Army today who are passing out drugs and medicines without the slightest educational qualification for that job, and that is what we want to break up.[52]

Rowland Jones, an attorney and representative of NARD, was the final individual to speak for pharmacy in the House hearings. He opened his comments with the statement that he represented 28,000 independent retail druggists. The focus of his comments was the inappropriate use of manpower. In addition to the position that the military would be better served by having pharmacists practice pharmacy rather than serve in the line or in some other non–health care position, Jones talked about the home front and the inappropriateness of removing professionals from where they were needed. He stated that "it is a reckless waste of manpower to put pharmacists into the armed forces in positions that others could better fill."[53] Jones concluded his testimony with a most intriguing accusation:

> This Committee has at its disposal voluminous evidence of dangerous malpractice which has existed in the Army down to this day. It is obvious that our national morale would be damaged were all of these facts to be released to the general public. They

are a matter for the consideration of the Military Affairs Committee in executive session.[54]

The bill was passed unanimously by the House on June 21.

The Senate Committee on Military Affairs held hearings on the Senate version of HR 997 on June 29, 1943. Norman T. Kirk was the new Army surgeon general. Robert Reynolds of North Carolina was the chair of the Senate committee. Carl Durham was the first to speak in support of his bill. He stated that there were only two purposes for the measure. The first was to give the men and women in the armed forces the same protection in the use of medicines enjoyed by civilians and the second was to place all procurement and distribution of medicines under the control of the corps of pharmacy officers.[55] In the questioning by the chair, Durham stated that twenty state legislatures had passed bills supporting the creation of the Pharmacy Corps.[56] Congressman Harve Tibbott, a Pennsylvania pharmacist, spoke next in support of the bill. L. S. Ray, the acting executive Secretary of the American Legion, reported that the American Legion had passed a resolution at its annual convention favoring the Pharmacy Corps bill and concluded, "I don't know of any bill that has been before us for a long time that has had stronger recommendation than this bill has had."[57]

Three representatives of pharmacy were scheduled to give formal statements: Kendig, Newton, and Jones. The formal statements were a repeat of the materials presented at the hearings before the House committee. Kendig offered new data that "by the end of 1942 some 10% of the pharmacists in the country were in the armed forces and 10% of the pharmacies of the United States had been closed."[58] Newton reported that enrollment in the colleges of pharmacy had dropped by 60 to 70 percent from 1941 to 1942. Senator Reynolds commented positively on the education of pharmacists, especially the mandatory internship before being licensed. He noted that several years earlier a gentleman in Washington, DC, identified as the chaplain of the Senate, was killed as a result of an improperly filled prescription.[59]

The final testimony of the hearing was given by General M. G. White of the surgeon general's office. He had no prepared statement but answered the questions put to him by the committee members. He was able to keep the questions away from the stated objective of centralizing pharmacy control and focused the discussion on whether the commissioning of seventy-two officers would provide any value—to anyone or anything other than the seventy-two involved.[60] General White took the position that the current Medical Administrative Corps was absolutely essential to the war effort and that the creation of the Pharmacy Corps would eliminate the MAC. This argument was successful, at least to the point where the discussion moved to questioning how the Pharmacy Corps could be established and the MAC not eliminated. White remarked that the "creation of a Pharmaceutical [*sic*] Corps probably won't do any harm. I don't consider it necessary for the proper administration of the Army."[61]

The hearings were concluded with the admonition to the pharmacy group to develop language in the bill that would allow the continuation of the Medical Administrative Corps. The Senate committee similarly directed General White to work with the pharmacy group to develop language that would allow for the creation of the Pharmacy Corps. Senator Gurney moved

> that the bill be reported out as we have just talked, and that the language receive the approval of the chairman of the committee, Senator Johnson and Senator Cabot Lodge, and when it does receive their approval it be reported on the floor of the senate as action of the full committee.[62]

The pharmacy and War Department representatives met and agreed to establish the Pharmacy Corps while leaving the MAC intact. Pharmacy insisted on the immediate transfer of sixteen officers to the new corps. The Army agreed, but insisted that forty-two nonpharmacist officers also be transferred. This seeming deadlock was broken when the pharmacy leaders were advised by both Senator Reynolds and Congressman Durham to take what they had. It might be impossible to gain the same ground after the Congress's summer recess.[63]

The Senate bill was passed by unanimous consent on July 3, 1943. The House accepted the amendments and passed the bill by unanimous consent on July 5. The final bill was sent to President Roosevelt for his signature on July 6 and was signed into law on July 12. The struggle for recognition was over. The Pharmacy Corps existed, and soon commissioned pharmacists would be moved to the new entity.

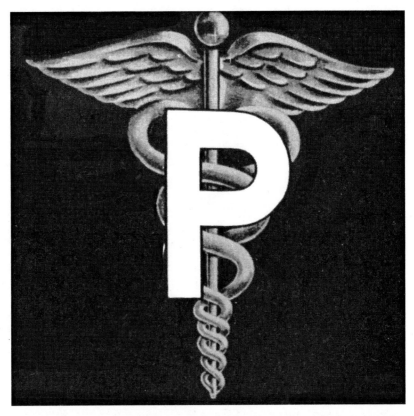

The insignia worn by officers in the Pharmacy Corps from 1943 until 1947 featured a gold caduceus with a letter "P" (for pharmacy) mounted in its center. (*Source:* Photo courtesy of the Lloyd Library and Museum.)

At the 1943 annual meeting of the American Pharmaceutical Association, H. Evert Kendig concluded the report of the Committee on the Status of Pharmacists in the Government Service:

> Your committee has now complied with your instructions through duly approved resolutions and, has brought about by Congressional action authorization for the establishment of a Pharmacy Corps in the United States Army. The organization of the Corps is a function and a duty of the Army. . . .
>
> While the tangible results of our success are valuable, the implications are very far reaching and of the utmost importance.

For the first time pharmacy has been recognized without restricting qualifications. Ultimately, this precedent will open all doors for pharmacy to participate on the proper basis where its services can be useful. That the profession will embrace with distinction its new opportunities is demonstrated by its past record of contributions to the public health and human welfare.[64]

With this conclusion, Kendig gave up the chair of the committee.

IMPLEMENTATION

New Jersey pharmacist Arthur Einbeck, a major in the inactive reserve of the Sanitary Corps, was appointed as the next chair of the Committee on the Status of Pharmacists in the Government Service. The attention of the committee in 1944 shifted to the status of pharmacists in the Navy and the implementation of the Pharmacy Corps in the Army.

A series of meetings occurred with Surgeon General of the Navy McIntyre and his staff to explore the creation of a separate pharmacy service in the Navy. In addition, pharmacy wanted the title of pharmacist's mate changed to better reflect the actual duties of the individual. McIntyre took the position that a separate pharmacy service was impractical but agreed with the objective of improving pharmaceutical services in the Navy. The tone of the meetings was described as "pleasant." Congressmen Durham and Rivers were part of the pharmacy group meeting with Admiral McIntyre and "were impressed with the Surgeon General's attitude" and promised that any legislation agreed to between pharmacy and the Navy could be passed that year.[65]

The experience with the Army was just the opposite. It recognized that the war was still on, but pharmacy was impatient to see the corps implemented. Exams for commissions to the new corps were not held until six months after the law was signed. At the request of the APhA committee, Durham contacted the Army general staff about the implementation of the Pharmacy Corps and was told that there were no barriers to Kirk's forming the corps "should he so desire." The APhA committee, again with Congressman Durham in attendance, met with officers in the surgeon general's office to discuss expectations and

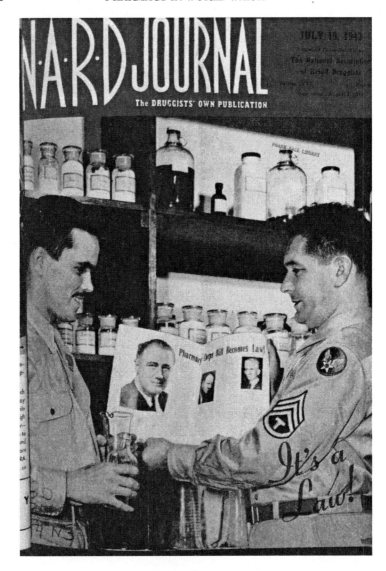

On July 12, 1943, Franklin Delano Roosevelt signed the Durham-Reynolds Bill establishing the Pharmacy Corps in the U.S. Army. This brought an official closure to a longstanding struggle for professional recognition between organized pharmacy and the Army. (*Source: NARD Journal* [1943] 65[July 19]:cover. Reprinted with permission. Photo courtesy of the Lloyd Library and Museum.)

implementation. There were a number of suggestions to make the continuing poor pharmaceutical services record of the Army public, including a letter to the president that a "mandate of Congress is being blocked."[66]

The status had not changed significantly a year later at the war-shortened APhA annual meeting. Pharmacy was still frustrated with the intransigence of the surgeon general and the lack of progress in forming the Pharmacy Corps. Pharmacy also recognized that the end of the war would require a major overhaul in the organization of the Army, including the Medical Department, and they wanted to be prepared to defend any gains made. Already there was a concern that the Pharmacy Corps would not be fully formed or survive the postwar reorganization.

Once again, the report on the relationship with the Navy was just the opposite. Ross McIntyre had forged a draft bill which provided that 20 percent of the commissioned officers be graduates of approved colleges of pharmacy and everything from "the specifications and procurement of drugs and medicines to the compounding and dispensing thereof will be the responsibility of those officers."[67]

The difference in the relationships of pharmacy with the Army and the Navy was of particular note. A positive dialogue started as early as 1916 with Secretary of the Navy Daniels. Surgeon General Stitt was a pharmacist himself, as well as a physician, and appeared to focus on the improvement of pharmaceutical services in his areas of responsibility. Finally, Surgeon General McIntyre also focused on the opportunities to improve pharmaceutical services. Consequently, the dialogue between the Navy and pharmacy never deteriorated to the point of hostility as it did with the Army. Pharmacy was satisfied with the increasing rank and responsibilities offered the pharmacists in the Navy and never took the position of forcing a separate corps.

Some of the most outstanding leaders of the profession were engaged in this struggle for professional recognition. Many of the presidents of the APhA were involved in the recommendations to continue the efforts of the Committee of Status of Pharmacists in the Government Service and the selection of the chair. Other pharmacy groups had their own committees and efforts to gain the same professional objective. A good indication of the level of leadership involvement is to consider that there were only six APhA committee chairs during the 1894-1943 period. Of these, three would become presidents of APhA and one an honorary president. The remaining two were presidents of NABP and AACP. Four of these six would win the Remington medal.*

As a direct result of his leadership role in the passage of the law securing the Pharmacy Corps, Kendig was awarded the Remington medal in 1944. In his Remington address Kendig rightfully acknowledged the truth that is the hallmark of so many human endeavors— the debt to those who have preceded:

> While I usually find myself in agreement with my good friend Dr. Swain, I cannot accept his version that the preceding committees or the preceding chairmen labored without results. It is true that the Pharmacy Corps objective was realized only in 1943, but there was a tremendous amount of constructive work done in the preceding years. These earlier efforts contributed much to a victorious conclusion, and fortuitous circumstances brought about a culmination of effort during my administration.[68]

---

*G. F. Payne, S. Hilton, and R. Swain were APhA presidents and E. F. Cook an honorary president. H. E. Kendig was the president of AACP, Winnie of NABP. Remington Medal winners were Cook (1931), Hilton (1935), Swain (1940), and Kendig (1944).

Chapter 7

The Military

We feel that the needs of the pharmacy branch—that is, the safe-guarding of and compounding of prescriptions, is now provided in our hospitals and our field installations.[1]

General Larry McAfee,
assistant to the U.S. surgeon general

The first definition of military pharmacy in the United States dates to 1777 when the duties of the apothecary general were "to receive, prepare, and deliver medicines, and other articles of his department to the hospitals and army."[2] Although the rank and office of the apothecary general later disappeared, the basic functions of receiving, preparing, and delivering medicines remained an integral part of military health care. Neither the Army nor the Navy had a separate pharmacy organization during World War II. Both branches provided pharmacy services as part of their medical program and both were opposed to the establishment of a separate pharmacy corps. Both branches used pharmacists and pharmacy technicians within their dispensaries, and neither considered pharmacists deserving of commissions to practice pharmacy.

During World War II the Army was the largest branch of the military. In 1941 the Army Air Corps was renamed the Army Air Force, which did not become a separate military service until 1947. The Army was responsible for the provision of all health services for itself and the Air Force. The Navy, smaller than the Army, also had responsibility for providing many services to the Marines, including health care. The Public Health Service provided health care for the Coast Guard and the Merchant Marine. In many respects, the military had a health care system that was not unlike health care delivery in the general population. Soldiers and sailors reported to sick call when ill and were diagnosed and prescribed for, just as if they were visiting a doctor's office in their hometowns. If a prescription was written, an individual would pick up the medication at one of the dispensaries. If hospitalized, services were provided to the wards by the hospital pharmacy. One major difference marking the military system from the civilian was the degree and extent of trauma from preparing for combat and combat itself. Thus, for the military, trauma was a far greater concern than the illnesses that dominated civilian practice. In civilian life, the system took care of illnesses and trauma of all—male and female, young and old. In the military the population was predominantly young men. Obstetrics, pediatrics, and geriatrics were specialties virtually unneeded in the military world. These realities had a large influence on the practice of pharmacy, especially in the types of pharmaceuticals needed and how they were delivered to the patients. In the military, there was no such institution as the local drugstore. The system was made up of infirmaries and dispensaries that were typically linked with the hospital. The dispensaries, like the hospital wards, would receive stock items from the central pharmacy.[3]

THE ARMY SUPPLY CATALOG

The Medical Department Supply Catalog was similar to a civilian wholesaler list but less flexible or inclusive. It provided a compilation of standard items that were centrally stored and distributed for the Army. Military hospitals and dispensaries in the United States could draw on the supply as needed; those overseas drew from an assigned central supply depot. Medical depots were established in Great Britain and in the Pacific to supply troops in the theaters of war.[4] In the Zone of the Interior, the continental United States, products not in the supply catalog could be obtained through local purchase; however, using the supply catalog was the preferred acquisition process. The supply catalog listed everything from drugs, chemical, stains, and biological products (Class 1) to veterinary equipment and supplies (Class 8) and field equipment and supplies (Class 9) (see Appendix V).

Supply levels were set depending on the size of the units that the hospital served. The allowance was typically stated as the allowance per 1,000 men per month. This control was developed to minimize hoarding of supplies in some units while others experienced shortages. The 1943 supply catalog, for example, established the allowance for bottles of 1,000 acetylsalicylic acid five-grain tablets at 5.75 per 1,000 men per month and bottles of 1,000 sodium bicarbonate five-grain tablets at 0.3976 per 1,000 men per month. Other products, such as smallpox vaccine, tetanus toxoid, and anthrax serum, were to be drawn as needed.[5]

The 1943 supply catalog for Class 1 products contained few items for patients with chronic problems such as diabetes or heart disease. Less than three dozen products were provided in oral tablet dose forms; most products were bulk standard items that could be used to compound the necessary finished dose forms. The oral tablets that were available were chiefly to treat the ills of a young healthy population, such as diarrhea, upset stomach, constipation, strains, and sprains. The catalog also contained a number of products that were not innocuous, such as mercuric cyanide and strychnine sulfate. The supply catalog was not strictly composed of ready-to-use tablets that could be dispensed by anyone who could read as represented by General McAfee at the 1942 House hearings on the establishment of a pharmacy corps.[6] An example of compounding skills was recalled by Myron Kirshner, a 1943 Temple graduate. He was drafted and assigned to an Army Air Force pharmacy. He compounded products, such as elixir of terpin hydrate and codeine, while stationed at Mitchell Field in Hempstead, New York. Terpin hydrate powder was dissolved in bulk alcohol in accordance with the *NF* formula. "The formula required the use of Oil of Orange which was not on the hospital list so we had to make our own." Peels from oranges obtained from the mess hall were removed, grated, and macerated in alcohol for twenty-four hours. The supernatant liquid was decanted and used to complete the *NF* formula for the cough syrup.[7]

What the supply catalog does not fully record is the type of pharmaceutical products that were of importance in the combat areas. These included improved anesthetics (such as sodium pentothal), Atabrine, blood plasma, morphine Syrettes, and, later, albumin, and the sulfas until their use fell out of favor after penicillin became available. Atabrine provided an example of how production was increased to meet military needs. In 1940, Winthrop Chemical Company produced approximately 5 million Atabrine tablets a year but was dependent on materials received from Germany's I. G. Farben, the patent holder. Research was successfully undertaken to develop the necessary steps for manufacture of the tablets—a complex process that used 1.5 tons of chemicals to make 100 pounds of Atabrine. In 1943 almost 1.8 billion tablets were delivered to the medical department; and over 2.5 billion were delivered in 1944.[8]

ARMY PHARMACY

Most materials stocked in the military pharmacy were obtained from one of the major medical supply depots which served a role similar to the wholesaler in civilian life.[9] For the most part physicians wrote prescriptions based on the official supply table. This use of an approved list of finished products, ingredients, and supplies provided an effective tool to discourage the use of proprietary products and more expensive products.

At the center of the medical supply chain was pharmacist Joseph G. Noh, a 1921 graduate of the University of Nebraska. Noh was too old to be drafted at the beginning of World War II. He had taught at the New Jersey College of Pharmacy and Purdue and served as the executive secretary of the Pennsylvania Pharmaceutical Association before joining McKesson and Robbins in 1929. In 1942 he enlisted in the Army, was given the rank of major, and was assigned the task of director of purchasing for all medical supplies and equipment for the Army. His department included five buying branches (biologicals; surgical and dental instruments; field hospital and laboratory equipment; textiles; and drugs and chemicals). By the end of the war Noh was promoted to lieutenant colonel and was responsible for purchasing for the first joint Army and Navy procurement of medical supplies; this assignment included procurement for the American Red Cross and International Aid.[10]

Counter to official testimony, compounding was the norm, at least at the large military posts. A number of products, such as cough syrups, boric acid solution, and ointments, were routinely compounded.

Where tablets would work, the use of capsules was discouraged. However, APC (acetylsalicylic acid, phenacetin, and caffeine) capsules were compounded, hand filled, and liberally supplied at sick call for all sorts of minor complaints. Prewar conditions also encouraged the use of high-alcohol elixirs since they were easy to compound and alcohol was both abundant and tax free to the military. This changed during the war as alcohol was a critical commodity in the war effort and liquid preparations were not as easy to transport as solid oral dosage forms were.

In many respects the practice of pharmacy in the military during the months leading up to Pearl Harbor was not that different from what was being practiced in drugstores around the county—with one exception. Army pharmacist F. E. Crowley wrote of the joys of practicing *"real* pharmacy," which he identified as using technical and professional knowledge as part of a well-functioning institution. The soda fountain, out-front merchandise, tobacco, and candy had no place in the military pharmacy.[11] A similar experience and sentiment was echoed in a 1944 paper describing the work of a military pharmacist in a stateside hospital. Harold H. Goldblum, a 1930 graduate of the Philadelphia College of Pharmacy, described the preparation of bulk orders for the wards and the afternoons spent in manufacturing such items as boric acid solution, elixir of terpin hydrate, and Brown Mixture. He added that he felt fortunate not having to deal with the fountain, cigarettes, or baby play pens, and noted the wonderful feeling of using professional skill "to bring health and normalcy back to the wounded men of this, the most terrible of all, wars."[12]

No information has been found on the number of Army pharmacies, either in the United States or overseas, that were operating during the war. The number of hospitals is also difficult to estimate because change was constant as training units were activated and sent overseas, and small hospitals merged into larger ones. There were also different types of hospitals, ranging from the large, named general hospitals in the United States, such as Walter Reed and Letterman, to the large, overseas numbered general hospitals, and the smaller portable surgical hospitals. Each of these facilities provided some level of pharmacy services.

Camp Butner, located near Durham, North Carolina, was developed as a training site for the Army in 1942. By the end of 1943, as the training facility for the 78th Infantry Division, the camp had 40,000 troops. The hospital pharmacy on the base was responsible for supplying the needs of the entire camp, which included thirty-five dispensaries. In the previous year the pharmacy had filled over 70,000 prescriptions and during the cold season had made over 5,000 gallons of cough syrup and more than 1 million cold tablets. There were at least three registered pharmacists and two technicians on the staff of the pharmacy.[13]

The inappropriate use of pharmacists in the military was a problem. A number of pharmacists in the armed forces were complaining that they were assigned to all kinds of duties that had nothing to do with pharmacy or even the broader medical field. After consultation with General McAfee, the American Pharmaceutical Association issued a bulletin to the secretaries of the state pharmaceutical associations, pharmaceutical publications, and the deans of the schools and colleges of pharmacy spelling out the number of pharmacists that the Army anticipated needing. The Army was planning for a force of 3.6 million men which would require 5,000 pharmacists to provide pharmacy services. The bulletin emphasized that as many of those pharmacists as possible who were drafted would be used in a professional capacity, and any shortfall would be made up with the use of graduates of a technical school. In addition, pharmacists were encouraged to apply for officer candidate schools and those with the necessary leadership and fitness for officer status would be recommended for selection. Those not selected for OCS would be assigned to medical department facilities with a specialist rating and serve in a noncommissioned grade. The bulletin concluded with an observation that should the Army double in size from General McAfee's estimate, it was likely that 10,000 pharmacists would be needed in the Army alone.[14]

PERSONAL EXPERIENCES

Pharmacists who entered the military had no guarantee that they would serve as pharmacists or even in the broader context of health services. Similarly, there was no guarantee of a commission, especially in the medical services. Some men preferred to opt for officer candidate school and went wherever they were assigned. Many men wanted to fly as commissioned pilots; others enlisted in the hopes of an assignment in a field that would more likely take them into combat. Many, perhaps most, wanted to practice their profession and tried to gain an assignment that would place them in health care. Melvin Gibson, a 1942 graduate of the University of Nebraska, combined courses in military sciences and field artillery with pharmacy. Upon graduation he was commissioned and ordered to active duty. He was able to delay long enough to take his state board examinations, the "last official connection with pharmacy" until his discharge in 1946. Gibson was awarded the Bronze Star for bravery on July 8, 1944, and was wounded in Dutch New Guinea on July 30. He was brought home; his war was over.[15]

No census has been found identifying how many pharmacists served in which service, in what capacity, or at what rank. In December 1944 the State Board of Pharmacy reported a survey of 228 Wisconsin pharmacists serving in the Armed Forces. Of the 136 respondents eighty-two (60 percent) were in the Army or Army Air Force and fifty-four in the Navy or Marines (40 percent). Seventy-five percent of the Army respondents reported that they were working in pharmacy or some related medical care role; 80 percent of those in the Navy reported similar assignments. In the Army, twenty-nine of the eighty-two were commissioned, holding ranks ranging from second lieutenant through lieutenant colonel; in the Navy, thirteen were commissioned, holding ranks ranging from ensign through lieutenant commander. The survey listed fifty-four specific duties, which included aviation psychologist, rifle marksmanship training, watch officer, LCT (landing craft-tank) captain, cryptographic technician, and bandsman. A number of those surveyed reported that they did not want pharmacy assignments in the service for some of the following reasons:

- Lack of satisfactory ratings
- Low esteem in which Army pharmacy is held
- Only for enlisted men
- Wants to get close to combat duty
- Pharmacy in the Army is not the way I want to practice
- Standing not what it should be
- No specific place in Army allotted to pharmacists

- No ratings high enough
- Not proper recognition
- Less chance for promotion[16]

John W. Mishler Jr. was not one of the respondents to the Wisconsin survey. A Nebraska native, he graduated from Creighton in May 1943. Mishler opted for enlistment in the Navy because it provided the opportunity to graduate and gain a commission as a line officer. He was assigned as officer in charge of USS *LCT 781* and proceeded from New Orleans through the Panama Canal to the Pacific. His LCT landed its tanks in the invasion of the Philippines on D-Day, October 20, 1944—the day before Douglas McArthur landed on Leyte.[17]

Whatever the reasons, many pharmacists were not engaged in pharmaceutical services or even in health care in the military. The military maintained that it would assign men to any task where manpower was needed. One example of this approach was evident in the eventual assignment of Alex Berman as a pharmacist in the Air Force. Berman, a 1937 graduate of St. John's, worked at a Walgreens store in New York City prior to entering the service in 1943. He told his story in poetic verses:

"HOW I BECAME A MILITARY PHARMACIST"

I Was an RPh. when called to serve
My Country. Did I not deserve
To practice my profession?
"No," said the Air Force—
"You'll take another course."

They marched me to the firing range,
Thrust a machine gun in my hands—
"We'll make you into a tail-gunner!"
I closed my eyes, the trigger squeezed—
Leaves and twigs fell from tops of trees.
A frightened officer seized my gun,
"This is not how a war is won!"
So, happily they let me be
A pharmacist in the American Army.[18]

Hundreds of pharmacists and pharmacy students were assigned to combat units, such as paratroopers, infantry, and aircraft crew, and had little to do with pharmacy or health care. Some men were assigned to pharmacy duty by the luck of the draw. Some men chose to do something in the military where they could receive a commission, and this decision led them to combat or to assignments in fields that had little to do with their specialized college training.

Charles Robinson graduated from Drake in 1940 and was in the Navy prior to Pearl Harbor. His first duty was in the Naval Recruiting Office in Des Moines, Iowa. He was serving as a pharmacist's mate on January 3, 1942, when the five Sullivan brothers enlisted. Robinson was later sent to midshipman school and commissioned. He received a Bronze Star for meritorious service in a Naval Combat Demolition Unit during the invasion of Southern France on August 15, 1944.[19]

Robert M. Atkins graduated from the University of Florida and passed his state boards in 1940. After several months of retail practice he was called into the service in October; commissioned as an infantry second lieutenant, he eventually served in the paratroops. He spent thirty-eight months in the Southwest Pacific and took part in three combat jumps, including the famous jump of February 16, 1945, on Corregidor Island.[20]

Exercise Tiger, a rehearsal for the invasion of Normandy, was carried out in Slapton Sands, England. Ray Gosselin, a 1943 Massachusetts College of Pharmacy graduate commissioned as a line officer in the Navy, was assigned as assistant gunnery officer on *LST 531*. *LST 531* was part of the exercise on April 28, 1944, when German patrol boats from Cherbourg attacked the American formation and hundreds of troops drowned. *LST 531* was hit and sunk; six of the nine officers were killed. Gosselin was awarded a Silver Star and Purple Heart for his part in the aftermath of the attack. He managed to get the wounded on a life raft and away from the sinking LST. The award citation stated,

> he then supervised the efforts of his men to keep the raft upright and navigated by the stars toward land. He was tireless in his efforts to keep the men on the raft awake and in possession of their faculties. At the end of six hours of all but complete submersion in the rough and ice-cold water, he succeeded in attracting the attention of a British destroyer which rescued all survivors.[21]

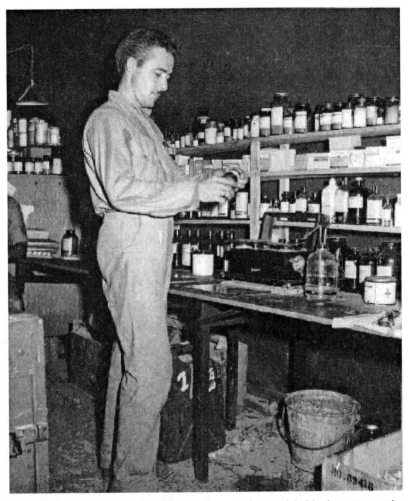

Pharmacist Mate J. W. Crutchfield checks over the stock in his drugstore under a tent in 1943 at a South Pacific base. (*Source:* Reprinted with permission from *Pharmacy in History* [1995] 37[4]. Photo courtesy of Drug Topics collection, American Institute of the History of Pharmacy.)

Thomas E. Griffin, a 1940 graduate of the University of Minnesota, enlisted in the Army, was sent to officer candidate school, and was assigned to the Medical Department as a supply officer. Griffin played a pivotal role in the delivery of medicines and supplies during the invasion of Normandy on June 6, 1944, for which he was awarded a Bronze Star for meritorious achievement in ground operations against the enemy. This involved a cargo ship with medical supplies for the planned invasion that was sunk before it reached England. On May 27 an emergency request was made for the "impossible" task of assembling eighty-four surgical units in four days for use in the impending invasion. The recommendation for Griffin's medal noted that each unit consisted of ninety boxes containing over 2,000 components. The request also included ninety-eight skids of medical maintenance units. Each unit consisted of 300 boxes and weighed over 2,300 pounds. In addition to packing materials for the invasion, Griffin was responsible for assembling five general hospitals and twenty-five Air Force dispensaries of twenty-five and fifty beds. The recommendation concluded that from "27 May 1944 to 1 June 1944, Thomas E. Griffin never left the job, working continuously day and night. So that on 1 June 1944 it was possible to report to the Chief of Service that the 'impossible' had been done."[22]

PHARMACY TECHNICIANS

The Army established its first school for pharmacy technicians in August 1939 at the Army Medical Center in Washington, DC. The justification for the school was to increase the skill level of the enlisted personnel who were filling prescriptions without any formal training. It was estimated that the Army needed at least 376 trained technicians for assignment to existing hospitals. The officer in charge of the training program was Second Lieutenant Glenn K. Smith, a 1936 graduate of Washington State and one of the first two pharmacists commissioned as pharmacists.[23]

Originally the pharmacy technician course was a nine-month program. Admission to the program was restricted to those enlisted personnel who were high school graduates or had considerable practical pharmacy experience. Each man had to be recommended by an officer who would attest to the individual's ability, character, and health. The men also had to have at least two years and eight months left in their current enlistment and were expected to reenlist. The technician would learn tasks that paralleled the duties of a civilian pharmacist. They included maintenance of drug stocks; manufacturing of galenicals and stock preparations; routine compounding and dispensing within the hospital; compounding and dispensing for outpatient dispensaries; and adequate record keeping.

Technician training focused on the practical applications rather than the theoretical background. Courses were required in chemistry, pharmaceutical arithmetic, and materia medica and therapeutics, as well as pharmaceutical compounding. The supply catalog provided a framework for what drugs to learn and preparations to compound. Since few galenicals were included in the catalog, the technician would be expected to compound them. A number of other medicines were either compounded or put up in individual doses for dispensing. While the technician would be supervised on the job, the supervisor might be a medical officer with limited experience in pharmacy, if any, rather than a graduate pharmacist.[24]

By early 1942 the need for pharmacy technicians had expanded in keeping with the needs of a growing Army. Six technician programs had been established: Army-Navy General Hospital, Hot Springs, Arkansas; Letterman General Hospital, San Francisco, California; Fitzsimmons General Hospital, Denver, Colorado; Army Medical Center, Washington, DC; William Beaumont General Hospital, El Paso, Texas; and Fort Sam Houston Station Hospital, San Antonio, Texas. The length of the training course had shrunk from the original nine months to ninety days. The course had a total of 468 hours of instruction with two hours daily devoted to lectures and five hours to laboratory work.

The ninety-day curriculum was a shorter version of the nine-month program. The major subjects were pharmaceutical arithmetic, chemistry, pharmacy, and therapeutics. The topic of pharmacy was broken into two major areas with the first covering general pharmacy and galenicals preparations and the second focusing on the military prescription. The technician was taught how to use and care for pharmacy instruments, tools, and supplies before learning how to compound *USP* and *NF* preparations. During the laboratory exercises approximately 125 different formulas were prepared. The student studied physical, therapeutic, and chemical incompatibilities and learned how to compound solutions, mixtures, capsules, powders, ointments, and suppositories. The combined pharmacy topics covered three-quarters of the total course time. At the end of the ninety days the technician received a recommendation for his new rank based on how well he had completed the course.[25] By June 1943, all of the Army "cram" schools for pharmacy technicians had been discontinued with the exception of the program at Fitzsimmons, perhaps because there were enough "ninety-day" grads.[26]

A number of the instructors in the Army's technician schools were pharmacists. Glenn K. Smith, a 1936 graduate of Washington State, was assigned to teach at the Army Medical Center in Washington, DC.[27] Other pharmacists teaching at the Army Medical Center in 1942 included Lieutenant Leon Rose (Columbia University, 1935), Lieutenant Henry M. Butler (George Washington University, 1933), and Lieutenant Robert Swan (Massachusetts College of Pharmacy, 1930). There were also at least three registered pharmacists with the rank of private assigned as laboratory assistants at the school, including Clarence Joyce (George Washington University, 1937), Thomas A. Moskey Jr. (University of Maryland, 1936), and Jack Snyder (Temple University, 1939).[28]

NAVY PHARMACY

Unlike the Army, the Navy had a tradition of pharmacy services. In 1866 the rank of surgeon's steward was changed to apothecary; when the Hospital Corps was established in 1898 the title pharmacist was substituted for apothecary. However, the naval rank of pharmacist was not an entry point for a civilian pharmacy-educated individual; instead it was a warrant officer rank that was earned after a number of years of service. During World War I, a number of chief pharmacists were temporarily commissioned but were returned to their permanent rank after the war. In 1940 any location assigned a medical officer had a naval pharmacy. This included at least forty dispensaries in naval hospitals and over 200 on board naval ships.[29]

The Hospital Corps was the enlisted component of the Medical Department of the Navy. All of the health care personnel, with the exception of commissioned physicians, were part of the Hospital Corps, including laboratory services, embalming administration, and pharmacy. The normal progression through the ranks started with hospital apprentice and, after sufficient time and experience, a promotion to pharmacist's mate. This grade created considerable confusion to civilians and others unacquainted with the naval ranks; traditionally a pharmacist's mate did not have to be a pharmacist or even provide pharmacy services. The major portion of the basic training in the Hospital Corps was for nursing which was done on war ships and many of the forward hospitals. Hospital Corps schools were initially maintained in Portsmouth, Virginia, and San Diego, California. As the wartime Navy grew, additional schools were established at Bainbridge, Maryland, Great Lakes, Illinois, and Farragut, Idaho. The total duration of the course was no more than eight weeks of instruction, which concentrated on nursing, first aid, and hygiene.

Most of the graduates of the schools were immediately assigned to hospitals, ships, or the Marines for duty. The exceptional students could achieve the rank of pharmacist's mate third class and be assigned to the specialty school at the naval hospital in Bethesda.[30] Pharmacists who entered the Navy were frequently allowed to bypass the early portion of the basic training and proceed immediately to the specialized training.[31] The Navy was suffering from a shortage of hospital corpsmen and determined that male nurses, pharmacists, chiropractors, dental technicians, Red Cross instructors, and firemen could skip recruit training if they had a rating of third class or above. Warren Higby graduated from Wayne State in 1942 and managed to take his state boards before enlisting in the Navy. He noted that he never marched, tied knots, rowed boats, slept in a hammock, or performed many of the other minutiae of basic training. Instead, he had a two-week course in bedside nursing.[32]

With the expansion of the military in 1941 the American Pharmaceutical Association asked the Navy if it would require as many as 1,500 registered pharmacists. The response was that 1,500 pharmacists who were physically qualified would be accepted at ranks ranging from pharmacist's mate second class through petty officers. Dwight Ferguson was one of the first pharmacists to see action in the opening days of the war. He graduated from the University of Florida in 1938 and enlisted in the Naval Reserve. In March 1941 he was called to active duty and assigned to the USS *Wakefield* in May. The ship was sent to Halifax where British troops were loaded and then headed south, but before reaching Cape Town, Pearl Harbor was attacked. The ship stopped in Bombay before heading for Singapore. On January 31, 1942, the *Wakefield* was attacked by the Japanese;

one bomb hit the sick bay, killing many and wounding Ferguson. Ferguson was sent to the Philadelphia Naval Hospital where he was the first combat casualty admitted.[33] By July 1943 the Navy had over 1,700 registered pharmacists in uniform.[34]

The Navy, like the Army, stated that minimal compounding was required to meet the needs of the service. This was undoubtedly true where space and expertise were almost absent, such as was the case in many of the ship infirmaries. However, compounding was an important function at many of the larger hospitals. At the Naval Dispensary in Washington, DC, 300 to 400 prescriptions a day were filled for Navy, Marine, and Coast Guard personnel and their dependents. The dispensary prepared bulk quantities of many products that were bought in ready-to-dispense form in civilian pharmacies. Examples included powders, such as foot powders and stomach powders, which were manufactured in lot sizes up to 200 pounds, and elixirs and syrups, which were prepared in ten-gallon quantities, and ointments in ten-pound quantities.[35] The dispensary at Great Lakes Training Center had sixteen registered pharmacists on staff by 1944 and manufactured over 1,000 pounds of fifty-five different ointments, 5,000 pounds of powders, 2,500 gallons of stock formulas, and 1.5 million tablets.[36] James Ellinger entered the Navy shortly after his 1943 graduation from the University of Washington and was eventually assigned to Treasure Island, California, working as a pharmacist. He recalled that almost everything they dispensed had to be compounded, including capsules of APC, APC with codeine, Whitefield ointment, elixir of terpin hydrate with codeine, and Brown's Mixture. At the request of the base dermatologist he compounded a number of formulations to treat the fungus infections with which South Pacific veterans were returning and, in the true naval tradition, called these formulations "gismos." One example was Gismo #13 for jock itch fungus which included phenol 1 percent, resorcin 2 percent, liquor carbonis detergens 2 percent, and calamine liniment qs 100.[37]

Many pharmacists were not assigned to large shore hospitals but to the ships and field hospitals. Every ship and station had a dispensary and each dispensary had a pharmacy, albeit small at times. The Navy attempted to distribute registered pharmacists so that every dispensary had at least one. In cases where there was no registered pharmacist, a graduate of the Hospital Corps training center would be used.[38]

Marvin S. Aaronson was a June 1944 graduate of the Philadelphia College of Pharmacy who immediately joined the Navy and received training at the naval hospital in San Diego, California. He was eventually assigned to the naval hospital in Philadelphia. The officer in charge of pharmacies wrote of Aaronson's duties and performance:

> His work consisted primarily of rendering pharmaceutical service that included the ordering, handling, preparing, storing, issuing and dispensing of chemicals, drugs, poisons, medicines, narcotics, compounding and dispensing of physicians prescriptions. Aaronson kept the records and made reports of the hospital's use, dispensation and consumption of alcohol, narcotics, whiskey, streptomycin, open purchase and the drugs on the United States Navy Supply Table.
>
> While in charge of manufacturing for the three pharmacies (Family Out Patient, Veterans Out Patient, U.S. Naval Hospital), he increased the efficiency of, designed and also established procedures for the production of pharmaceutical preparations used in the treatment of patients.[39]

PHARMACY-CHEMISTRY TECHNICIANS

At the beginning of the war there was a single advanced training program located at the Naval Medical Center in Bethesda, Maryland. Advanced training was available to those men who had been promoted through the ranks to pharmacist's mate or to civilian pharmacists who entered the service as a pharmacist's mate. The nine-month course included over 1,400 hours of classroom lectures and laboratory instruction. Subjects included chemistry, pharmaceutical arithmetic, operative pharmacy, dispensing, materia medica, and toxicology. The texts used for the courses included the *Handbook of the Hospital Corps*, the *United States Pharmacopoeia XII*, and the *National Formulary VII*.[40] Upon successful conclusion of the course the pharmacist's mate received his certificate as a pharmacy-chemistry technician.

NAVAL SUPPLY TABLE

In 1940 the main naval supply depot was located at the Naval Yard in New York City with subsidiary depots on Mare Island, California, and a third in the Philippines. In 1940 the Naval supply catalog was similar to the Army's version: Part I contained general medical supplies and equipment (i.e., expendable and nonexpendable drugs, chemicals, biologicals); Part II contained supplies for field medical units; and Part III contained supplemental items. In 1940 the supply catalog consisted of fewer than 250 preparations including 159 *USP* items, eleven *NF* items, and fifty-eight biologicals and reagents.[41]

A Navy compendium of pharmaceuticals provides a number of formulas in use including the ubiquitous APC capsules (aspirin 0.195 g, phenacetin 0.130 g, citrated caffeine 0.032 g in a No. 1 capsule shell). The same compendium lists articles that the pharmacist could be called upon to compound, especially aboard ship. The items ranged from cleaning formulas (sodium perborate, sodium borate, trisodium phosphate) to face powder (starch, purified talc, magnesium carbonate, perfume) and shampoo (oil of myrcia, oil of pimento, oil of orange, potassium carbonate, soft soap, glycerin, alcohol, distilled water). The compendium still listed a quinine hair lotion (quinine sulfate, perfumed spirit, bay rum, alcohol, glycerin, rose water) that was probably not compounded because of the general shortage of quinine.[42]

PUBLIC HEALTH SERVICE:
COAST GUARD/MERCHANT MARINE

Congress formed the Marine Hospital Service, the precursor agency for the Public Health Service, in 1798. From its inception the objective of the Marine Hospital Service was to provide health care to American merchant seamen and the Revenue-Cutter Service.[43] This mission continued when the Coast Guard was formed in 1919 by combining the Revenue-Cutter Service and the Life-Saving Service.[44]

During peacetime the Coast Guard is a part of the Treasury Department but in time of national emergency it becomes part of the Navy.

By executive order, President Roosevelt transferred the Coast Guard to the Navy Department on November 1, 1941. During the initial stages of the war the Coast Guard remained responsible for training cadets and officers of the United States Maritime Service; on August 31, 1942, the Maritime Service was transferred to the War Shipping Administration.[45]

Most merchant shipping was in war zones as supplies were carried across the Atlantic and Pacific Oceans to American and Allied troops. Enemy submarines were pressing close to both coasts and sinking ships within sight of the shore. (According to Merchant Marine records 169 ships were sunk off the Atlantic coast of the United States and twenty-seven on the Pacific Coast.)[46] At the beginning of the war most merchant ships carried a Public Health Service medicine chest, but none of the ships had a doctor or a trained hospital corpsman on board. The Maritime Service did not include a Hospital Corps as the Navy did. The Public Health Service developed a training program for pharmacist's mates for the Merchant Marines; the first class started on December 7, 1942, and graduated the following March.

The course was given at the U.S. Marine Hospital Corps School at Sheepshead Bay, Brooklyn, New York. The course included three weeks of basic training in seamanship followed by three months (ninety days) of classroom and laboratory training. Courses included emergency treatment and minor surgery, hygiene and sanitation, and nursing and pharmacy. The goal was to train the man to operate in an independent duty on a cargo ship or tanker at sea.[47] After graduation the corpsman received twelve weeks of supervised experience before being assigned to a ship.[48] An early lecture emphasized the nature of the war emergency for the would-be pharmacist's mates:

> In so called "normal times," it would be against all the accepted principles of medical ethics to be teaching Pharmacist's Mates diagnoses and treatments. However, these are not normal times— we are at war, and a goodly number of you will be on board a ship and will be expected to carry on alone the duties of a ship's doctor.[49]

Instructors for the school were drawn from the Public Health Service. Lacking a cadre of an existing hospital corps, civilians with qualifications in health care were recruited for the first class. Charles Bliven, an ensign in the Maritime Service and the assistant dean at George Washington University College of Pharmacy was placed in charge of the course on pharmacy.[50] In 1944 George Archambault, on leave from the Massachusetts College of Pharmacy, assumed the post of chief pharmacist at the United States Marine Hospital in Boston. Among his other duties he provided the lectures on pharmaceutical mathematics and essentials of compounding. In his lectures he recognized the importance of the roles of the seamen and urged caution:

> The Medical Officer in charge of this hospital has informed me that you men are to be "Doctor, Pharmacist, and Nurse" to your shipmates once your vessel leaves port. This places a serious responsibility on your shoulders. In some instances, where your ship is far from the outpost of civilization or where communication channels are unavailable for war reasons, important decisions must be made by you alone. . . . My particular assignment is not to teach you the profession of pharmacy. The essentials of the profession that are considered necessary for you to master have already been presented to you at Sheepshead Bay or at Columbia. My task is to review some of the "highlights" of the course already presented you, with the viewpoint of reminding you to "play safe."[51]

The Public Health Service publication *Ship's Medicine Chest and First Aid at Sea* was used as the standard reference for both the Coast Guard and Merchant Marine. One of the items in the publication was a list of medicines and supplies that should be available in each ship. Operations regulation No. 67 of the War Shipping Administration updated the minimum standard list of drugs, chemicals, and surgical supplies in July 1943 and again in March 1944. The supply list was based on a seventy-five-man crew for a three-month voyage, and contained short notes on the use and administration of most items. Among the items in the medicine chest were six bottles of 100 five-grain acetylsalicylic acid tablets, one 200 cc bottle of boric acid, one bottle of 1,000 tablets of opium, and olycyrrhiza compound for coughs. Ships with a doctor or a graduate of the Hospital Corps School were authorized to carry blood plasma and penicillin. The medicine chest also contained 100 sets of venereal disease (VD) prophylactic kits.[52]

In 1942 the Coast Guard was rapidly adding officers and seamen. The service was finding it difficult, however, to train the necessary support personnel. The courses for hospital corpsmen were capable of handling only forty trainees in each ninety-day cycle. The Navy had used Columbia University College of Pharmacy as a training site for hospital corpsmen during World War I and so the Coast Guard, now under the command of the Navy, approached Columbia to contract as a training site for its hospital corpsmen. The time interval between the initial contact and the arrival of students was a mere ten days. In that time housing was found at a nearby YMCA and all necessary arrangements for facilities at the school arranged.

On May 17, 1942, the first group of 200 Coast Guard men arrived at Columbia to begin their training. The course of instruction at Columbia mirrored the course at New London, Connecticut. The duration was ninety days, with most of the instruction delivered by Coast Guard personnel. The *United States Navy Hospital Corps Handbook* was the course text and instruction was in first aid, chemistry, and pharmacy. The last group of men graduated in February 1944; in the twenty-one months of operation almost 1,200 men had completed the course.[53]

In his history of Columbia College of Pharmacy, Dean Ballard summarized the training given to the hospital corpsmen of the Coast Guard. His words provide an insight to the training given by all of the Armed Forces:

> If measured by customary standards, the instruction in all branches excepting first aid was extremely superficial, but it served the urgent need for men who had sufficient knowledge of what to do and how to do it in giving emergency treatment.[54]

A number of pharmacists also served in the Coast Guard and Merchant Marines. Aaron Brodski, a 1939 graduate of the Brooklyn College of Pharmacy, enlisted in the Coast Guard in 1942 and served *on LST 176* as a pharmacist's mate in the D-Day invasion of Normandy.[55] Max Clayton, a 1939 graduate of Ohio State, also chose the Coast Guard. After his basic training he was assigned to teach new pharmacist's mates in New London. In early 1943 he was assigned to the U.S. Coast Guard Landing Craft Infantry (Large) Flotilla Four/Ten and took part in the landings in Salerno and Normandy.[56]

Civilians also became an important part of the Coast Guard service. The total size of the service had been restricted by Congress. As the Coast Guard was assigned duties in the combat areas it was essential to develop a method of protecting harbor facilities on the coasts and a Coast Guard Temporary Reserve was created. These individuals were civilian volunteers who agreed to donate twelve hours a week without pay or veteran status. They did wear regular Coast Guard uniforms and had the responsibilities and prerogatives of the service. Linwood Tice, dean of the Philadelphia College of Pharmacy, was one of the volunteers on the East Coast. He commanded a thirty-eight foot picket boat on the Delaware Bay transferring military ship pilots and convoying munitions-laden barges on the Delaware River. He was discharged with the rank of ensign at the end of the war.[57] In Seattle a group of forty pharmacists manned the Port Sick Bay. Two men were on duty in two shifts, seven days a week. Their duties included laboratory tests, first aid, immunizations, diagnosis of gonorrhea, and physical examinations as well as filling prescriptions.[58]

WOMEN IN THE ARMED SERVICES

At the end of 1942 the military started recruiting an increasing number of women. The expansion of women's services was justified on the basis of freeing young men for duty overseas. The Women's Army Auxiliary Corps (WAAC) was the largest service and was originally only an auxiliary unit and technically not part of the Army. This was changed in September 1943 when it became the Women's Army Corps (WAC), part of the regular Army. The Navy's WAVES (Women Appointed for Voluntary Emergency Service) were the Women's Reserve of the Navy Reserve and the SPARS (*Semper paratus*—"always ready"—the motto of the Coast Guard) were the Women's Reserve of the Coast Guard. In a meeting with the American Council on Education, representatives of the women's services outlined their individual needs and requirements. Initially, only the WAVES and SPARS identified a need for pharmacists.[59]

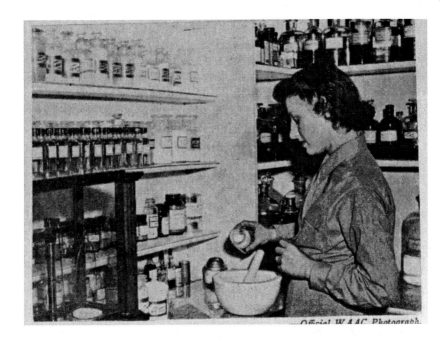

The Women's Army Auxiliary Corps (WAAC), formed in 1942, changed its name to the Women's Army Corps (WAC) in 1943. The military was interested in recruiting women for service in the States, thus freeing men for overseas duty. Helen Wetterstroem, a 1937 graduate of the Cincinnati College of Pharmacy, enlisted and trained at Fort Des Moines, Iowa. (*Source: NARD Journal* [1943] 65[March 15]:404. Reproduced with permission. Photo courtesy of the Lloyd Library and Museum.)

The first class of WAVES in the history of the Hospital Corps reported to the San Diego Naval Hospital in January 1943. The course that the women followed was shorter than the men's, largely because almost all of the women were college graduates. At least two of the original class were pharmacists—Ruth Peterson, a graduate of the Oregon State College, and Verna Herbison, a graduate of the University of Washington.[60] In November 1945, *American Druggist* wrote about eight pharmacists who were serving in the WAVES at St. Albans Hospital on Long Island, New York, and the naval hospital at Bethesda. The article concluded with a Navy statement that the women's profession "has made it possible for them to take a valuable part in upholding the motto of the Medical Department of the U.S. Navy— 'to keep as many men at as many guns as many days as possible.' " The article noted that there were a total of twenty-seven women pharmacists in the WAVES.[61]

The WAACs started recruiting pharmacists in February 1943.[62] In June 1944 the Army surgeon general authorized a drive for 200 pharmacists and 200 pharmacist's aides to join the Women's Army Corps, thus freeing men who could then be reassigned overseas. The duties of the pharmacist included compounding and dispensing medicines as directed by physicians, maintaining prescription records, and safe-keeping poisons, alcohol, and habit-forming drugs. The woman would receive a comparable rank to the man that she was replacing, technical sergeant, depending on her abilities and existence of vacancies in her assigned organization.[63] Margaret LaBrune Mixon, a 1941 graduate of the University of Nebraska, enlisted in the WACs in August 1944 and was sent to Fort Des Moines for her basic training before being assigned to LaGarde General Hospital in New Orleans as a pharmacist.

Like their male counterparts, women pharmacists were not necessarily assigned to duty in the pharmacy. Stephanie Podzunas Riopel, a Massachusetts College of Pharmacy graduate, was commissioned in the WAACs and was assigned to the training command. Paula Towle was a graduate of the University of California–San Francisco. After working in both retail and hospital pharmacy she enlisted in the WAVES in 1943. She was commissioned and served as a line officer in the Bureau of Naval Personnel.[64]

THE CORPSMAN AND THE MEDIC

Both the Army and the Navy assigned men with specialized training to accompany combat troops. The Army title was medic; the Navy was corpsman. Despite the different titles, the tasks were the same—to go in harm's way and provide first aid as soon after a man was wounded as possible. Not all of the medics or corpsmen served under combat situations, but many did and they learned to use morphine Syrettes, plasma, and sulfa under fire. Much of the credit for saving the lives of so many wounded men can be attributed to the quick responses and care that these men provided under actual battle conditions.

Carl C. Baker, a 1940 graduate of the Indianapolis College of Pharmacy, enlisted in the Navy in 1942 and was sent to Great Lakes for training. In early 1944 he and hundreds of other hospital corpsmen were loaded into LSTs in Bayone, New Jersey; they sailed to Scotland and then England. He took part in what would become known as Exercise Tiger, an aborted training landing for the invasion of France. Later, his LST made three trips to the invasion beaches of Normandy landing supplies and bringing back wounded German prisoners of war. Baker was sent back to the States and assigned to duty with the Fleet Marine Medical Service; the Navy provided health care for the Marines. Assigned to the invasion on Iwo Jima, he landed on the beach the third day of the invasion to set up a field hospital.[65]

MEMORIAL

A measure of the danger that many pharmacists faced in their military career is the number of individuals who were killed, wounded, or imprisoned in a prisoner-of-war camp. A least 131 men died during their time in the service; most of them were either killed in action or died as a result of wounds (see Appendix VI).

Paul Stanley Frament graduated from the Albany College of Pharmacy in June 1939. He enlisted in the U.S. Navy after Pearl Harbor and, in January 1942, reported for training as a pharmacist's mate. Frament was posted to the First Marine Division that was being organized for the Solomons invasion. He landed in the first invasion on August 7, 1942. On November 3, 1942, Frament's battalion engaged in an offensive action. During the fighting he rushed to a Marine and tended his wounds while ignoring the Japanese snipers shooting at him. Later in the battle he ignored mortar fire to aid other wounded men and in doing so was knocked unconscious by a close explosion. He was evacuated to the rear, but the following morning secured his own release and returned to his unit. On November 10, Frament, again under fire, tended the wounded. Finally he had to be evacuated because of exhaustion. Two days later he was wounded by naval gun-

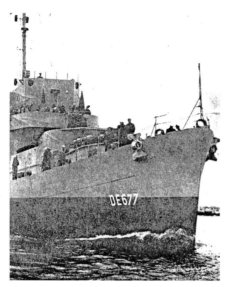
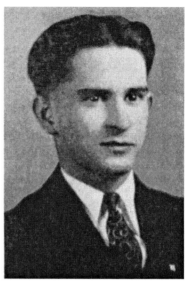

At least 131 pharmacists and pharmacy students died during their military service. Paul Stanley Frament, a 1939 graduate of Albany College of Pharmacy, enlisted in the Navy immediately after Pearl Harbor and was assigned to the Marines First Division. He died of wounds on Guadalcanal. Awarded the Silver Star for bravery, a destroyer escort was named in his honor. The ship was commissioned by his mother on August 15, 1943. Paul Stanley Frament, dead before the age of twenty-five, was one of the most highly decorated pharmacists in the U.S. Navy. (*Source: PostScript* [2002] 13[1]:2-3. The Alumni Magazine of the Albany College of Pharmacy. Reprinted with permission.)

fire and died on November 19, 1942. Frament was posthumously awarded the Silver Star for bravery. The Navy announced that a new destroyer escort, *DE 677,* under construction in Quincy, Massachusetts, would be named the USS *Frament.* The ship was commissioned by his mother on August 15, 1943. Paul Stanley Frament, dead before the age of twenty-five, was one of the highest decorated pharmacists in the U.S. Navy.[66]

Chapter 8

Epilogue: The Returning Veterans

FOR THE DURATION AND SIX MONTHS

May 8, 1945. August 14, 1945. The long-awaited days marking the end of the war finally arrived with the unconditional surrender of Germany in May and Japan in August. For the millions who served in the military it signaled a countdown to the time when they would once again be civilians. The Selective Service and Training Act, as amended after Pearl Harbor, established the limits for military service to be the duration of the war plus six months.[1] The trickle of men being discharged would soon turn into a flood. A 1939 graduate of the Cincinnati College of Pharmacy, August Elsener, recalled his assignment of detached duty making eight round trips on troop ships crossing the Atlantic. After the cessation of hostilities, the trips to the States were with returning servicemen and sometimes war brides and their children. On these trips

> passing the statue of Liberty was the most moving experience. All of the GIs crowded to the port side to see her and refused to leave even when the ship listed. The war-hardened men were crying like babies, and the captain had to suffer with the list, for the men were coming home.[2]

With the war over in Europe, many men were calculating how soon they might be demobilized. Initially a point system identified those to be separated. A soldier needed eighty-five points, calculated as follows:

- *Service credit*—one point for each month of Army service since September 16, 1940 [the date of enactment of the Selective Service Act].

- *Overseas credit*—one point for each month served overseas since September 16, 1940.
- *Combat credit*—five points for *each* award for service after September 16, 1940. Awards were those for bravery such as the Distinguished Flying Cross and the Silver Star; for participation in combat such as Bronze Service Stars; and Purple Heart Medals.
- *Parenthood credit*—Twelve points for each child under the age of eighteen, up to a limit of three children.[3]

The point system did not apply to officers or to enlisted men in critical military occupational specialties, such as radar, communications, and cryptographics. It also did not apply to officers who had the added requirement of "military necessity." The point system was not completely satisfactory, especially after the surrender of Japan; so the system was replaced by a length-of-service policy.[4]

Manpower issues remained a constant source of discussion throughout the war. Even in 1945 there was still a question about the severity of the shortage of pharmacists. Leslie Barrett of the University of Connecticut challenged the reality of the shortage during the 1945 District I meeting of the boards and colleges. He pointed out that there were times when physicians and nurses were not to be had, but challenged whether there was ever a time when someone could not get a prescription filled or medicine could not be obtained because of a lack of a pharmacist. There was some concern that the end of the war would result in a flood of applicants to pharmacy schools repeating the problems of oversupply that existed after World War I. The solution suggested was to limit enrollments in the colleges and to accept only the best of applicants.[5]

The end of the war brought issues and challenges to pharmacy; Charles Gilson, a member of the NARD executive committee, identified several. His first concern was the possibility that pharmacy technicians trained in the various military schools would seek licensed status on the basis of their military service. The return of 14,000 registered pharmacists was seen as both an immediate answer to the manpower shortage and as the potential for a glut of new stores.[6] College enrollments increased due to the returning students and were amplified by servicemen who wanted to take advantage of the GI Bill of Rights. Rationing and shortages quickly disappeared as the factories turned from producing war materials to the civilian goods that had been missing for the duration of the war.

Some men did not come home to work. Some found careers that they preferred to follow instead of pharmacy. Some came home physically or mentally unable to resume their lives in pharmacy. Some did not come home at all; as already noted at least 131 pharmacists and pharmacy students were killed during their military service. In one case a state board took special notice. The Wisconsin Board posthumously bestowed the rank and dignity of Registered Pharmacist on John Peter Shatrwka of Kenosha, a 1941 graduate of the University of Wisconsin who was killed in action.[7]

BACK TO WORK

In September 1945 an editorial in *American Druggist* proclaimed that drugstore operations should return to normal within six months, but there would be new challenges as well. The first challenge would be competition for the consumers' dollars when products unavailable during the war would compete for the disposable income that had bought drugstore items during the war. Another challenge would come from grocery stores, supermarkets, and variety stores taking on product lines traditionally claimed by drugstores. Druggists were encouraged to emphasize the unique character of the drugstore and noted that "super-markets may offer cold cream, but no woman likes to get her glamour in the same bag with potatoes."[8]

Many of the state boards were inclined to help the returning veterans as much as they could while still maintaining standards. A number of men finished school prior to leaving for the military but had been unable to take their board exams. Frequently this was because of regulations requiring completion of the intern year prior to sitting for one or both parts of the exam. Neil Schwartau experienced this. A 1943 graduate of the accelerated program at the University of Minnesota, he immediately enlisted in the Navy, was commissioned as an ensign, assigned to an LST, and sent to the South Pacific. A fungal infection colloquially called "jungle rot" was one of the major health problems in the area. There was no cure, but his chief pharmacist's mate called his attention to the use of yellow oxide of mercury reported in a medical journal. There was no such product in Naval stores, so Schwartau compounded one when he found that the ship had mercury bichloride for use in sterilization and the laundry had lye (sodium hydroxide). When he returned to civilian life, he was short the full experience needed to sit for the state board exams. During the board interview to determine if any military experience might compensate for the missing time, the compounding story was shared and the board allowed him to take the exam.[9]

All returning veterans were guaranteed their old jobs by the Selective Training and Service Act. The veteran did not have to meet higher standards than existed when he had left for the service.[10] Much had changed in the drugstore in the years since the beginning of the war. In response to manpower shortages operating hours had been drastically shortened, in many cases to less than ten hours a day. Many of the merchandising lines had disappeared due to product shortages and the prescription business had increased in size and profitability. New medicines were available and compounding was decreasing as manufacturers provided more products in ready-to-dispense dosage forms.

Concern arose that many pharmacists returning from the service would rush to open new stores, especially since the GI Bill provided veterans with low interest loans to buy or establish a new business. An influx of new stores was seen as a potential threat to established stores.[11] Writing in the *Carolina Journal of Pharmacy,* H. C. McAllister, secretary of the state board, stated that it "could not be demonstrated that there is a valid need for opening more drugstores" in North Carolina.[12] The number of pharmacies did increase in the postwar period, growing from 49,311 in 1946 to 51,263 in 1949.[13]

Refresher courses for the returning service man who had not practiced pharmacy or been engaged in some health services capacity in the military were planned. Several colleges discussed the type of course and format for programs that ran from several weeks to up to a year. The Wisconsin State Board of Vocational and Adult Education developed an outline for a brush-up course in pharmacy. The 1,000-hour program covered topics such as sources of technical information (100 hours), *USP* and *NF* changes (200 hours), and prescription problems (200 hours). The total cost for the course to the student was estimated at sixty-three dollars.[14]

HOSPITAL PHARMACY

While much of the focus of pharmacy leaders during the war was on retail practice, hospital pharmacy was gaining increased recognition. The APhA Sub-Section on Hospital Pharmacy became a separate organization, an affiliate of APhA, with the formation of the American Society of Hospital Pharmacists in 1942. By the end of the war ASHP had approximately 500 members.[15] Fischelis and Fiero had noted in their 1943 publication that 3,000 pharmacists were engaged in hospital practice in 1940.[16] This number had grown to 4,000 by mid-1944; the growth was presumed to come from pharmacists leaving retail practice.[17] In 1945, Henry Burlage of the University of North Carolina School of Pharmacy reported a survey of returning servicemen to determine what kinds of training would be of interest.

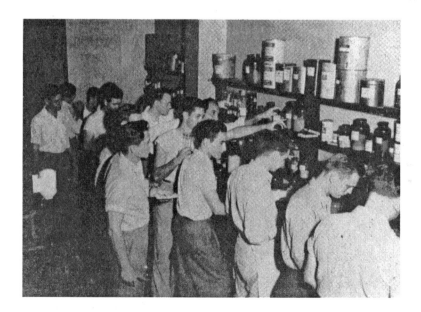

"The men came back from the service and they had families, and all they did was study. They were really working." The enrollment at colleges of pharmacy dramatically increased with veterans using the GI Bill. The dispensing laboratory at the University of Florida was bursting at the seams with the influx. (*Source:* Wanda Cowart Ebersole in the University of Florida 75th Anniversary Calendar. Reprinted with permission.)

Burlage noted that there was a considerable interest in hospital pharmacy and that this came as a "distinct surprise" and offered the observation that, if the findings were representative on a national basis, a sizable group of GIs "would like to take up this branch of professional service."[18]

The *American Professional Pharmacist* surveyed hospital pharmacists in preparation for the Pharmaceutical Survey (the Elliott Report). The survey was sent to approximately 3,000 pharmacists in August 1946; 334 responses were received. Over half of the responding hospitals (184) said that a pharmacist was required to be in attendance at all times and 101 said that a pharmacist only had to be present most of the time. Almost 60 percent of the hospitals hired only one full-time pharmacist, but a few had hired six or more. Female pharmacists were almost 35 percent of the pharmacists employed in the hospitals. The survey also noted that over 10 percent of the hospital pharmacies were supervised by the chief resident physician or the superintendent of nurses.[19]

GI BILL

Remembering the social disruption caused by the return of servicemen after WWI, many wanted to avoid a larger problem after WWII. In 1918 the problem centered on absorbing the discharged veterans into civilian jobs and finding adequate housing. On July 28, 1943, President Roosevelt raised the issue of what to do about veterans' benefits, but little was accomplished until the American Legion began a national campaign for comprehensive legislation.[20] William Randolph Hearst, with his national chain of newspapers, was a major supporter of the American Legion's campaign. The Servicemen's Readjustment Act, better known as the GI Bill of Rights and passed unanimously by both the House and Senate, was signed into law on June 22, 1944, less than three weeks after D-Day in Normandy.

The GI Bill of Rights contained provisions dealing with the expansion of the Veterans Administration hospitals and the health care benefits for those disabled during military service. The bill also contained benefits never before accorded to veterans. These included unemployment benefits, which provided an allowance of twenty dollars a week for up to fifty-two weeks. The loan portion of the bill provided a guarantee for up to 50 percent of a loan, or a maximum of

$2,000, toward the purchase of a home or business. The maximum interest on the mortgage could not exceed 4 percent per year. The loan could also be used to purchase machinery or tools needed by the veteran as part of his occupation.[21] The provision that allowed the purchase of a business was limited to two years after discharge or two years after the termination of the war, which encouraged those interested in purchasing a pharmacy to do so relatively quickly.[22]

The GI Bill also allowed those whose education had been impeded, delayed, interrupted, or interfered with to receive educational benefits. Frank Hines, administrator of veterans' affairs, noted that the law provided for anyone not over the age of twenty-five who had his education interrupted or delayed.[23] Educational benefits could be used for refresher courses, vocational training, and undergraduate or graduate courses as long as the eligibility and performance standards were met. The veteran had to have served at least ninety days and been discharged under conditions other than dishonorable. The GI Bill would provide for tuition, books and supplies, and fees for one year. If the student-veteran met the standards of the educational institution, additional periods of training were authorized. The maximum benefit was four years or a time equal to the time spent in the military between September 16, 1940, and discharge. In addition, the veteran received fifty dollars per month living allowance; the amount was increased to seventy-five dollars per month if the veteran had dependents. Veterans had to begin the educational program within two years of discharge and complete it within seven years of the end of the war.[24] The time limit for educational benefits, like the loan benefits, meant that many wanted to start school as quickly as possibly to get maximum benefits from the GI Bill.

Freas Brittingham returned to pharmacy school on the GI Bill far more experienced than when he left to enter the service. He recalled being drafted in 1943 and after basic training being assigned to the 31st Division in New Guinea in preparation for the invasion of the Philippines. He gave up his rifle for a medic's kit in time for the push from Mindanao. He was awarded a Bronze Star for heroism for moving forward to treat casualties under fire in front of the American lines on May 6, 1945.[25] He was awarded a Silver Star for bravery for his actions on June 5. The citation read in part that a soldier was severely wounded and that Brittingham voluntarily and with complete disregard for his own safety, went back to the stricken man and calmly removed his clothes and administered first aid. Then, although the wounded man outweighed him, he shouldered him alone, since it was impossible for others to help, due to the narrowness of the ridge, and unwaveringly carried him to the rear despite the fact that several men were killed along the trail that he was following.[26]

He graduated from the University of Missouri–Kansas City in 1951.[27]

University administrators were concerned about the nature of these new students. The students were more mature, focused on why they were in school and on finishing as quickly as possible. They were willing to tolerate crowded conditions but wanted classes that were practical and realistic rather than theoretical.[28] M. Joe Hardwick returned to West Virginia University "married and under the GI Bill" after serving with the Navy:

> We walked because there were not many cars. We stayed home because there was no money to spend. We studied because we had the feeling that we were committed and that the people paying the bills were watching and there was not a second chance. The general attitude on campus was not one favorable to returning veterans in general because they were older, married, and more apt to respond with what was on their minds.

Hardwick graduated in 1948.[29]

The pharmacy world had mixed feelings about the educational components of the GI Bill. As early as December 1945 editorials began appearing in state journals warning about the potential glut of pharmacy students and the inability of the colleges to handle the influx. Under the headline "Too Many Pharmacy Students!!!" Dean Rudd of the Medical Collge of Virginia raised the issue of too many pharmacists becoming a glut on the market and driving wages and working conditions as low as they were after World War I.[30] In an unsigned editorial, "Too Many Students?", the *Carolina Journal of Pharmacy* stated that the current facilities and faculty were insufficient to meet the swollen enrollment and suggested that something be done to limit the class size to a level more in keeping with the needs of the state.[31]

In January 1945 the total enrollment for the colleges of pharmacy was 3,349; almost 50 percent (1,599) women.[32] In April 1946 the American Association of Colleges of Pharmacy provided an enrollment tabulation (see Table 8.1) of sixty-five colleges as of the winter 1945-1946. It reflected the impact of returning veterans who comprised almost 50 percent of all students.[33] Many veterans returned to the point where their studies had been interrupted, but others were just beginning their college careers. The 1945-1946 data showed another postwar impact, namely the increased enrollment of men eligible for the draft. George Benson of Seattle was one of those whose college career was interrupted, and he returned to school changed by his military training and experiences. He was a student at the University of Washington before enlisting in the Navy in 1942. After basic training he was assigned first as a pharmacist's mate in the Pacific but in 1944 was ordered to Midshipmen's School at Columbia University. After graduation and commissioning he was assigned to the USS *Frederick Funston* for the landing of the Third Marine Division on Iwo Jima. Benson recalled being the officer of the deck on February 23, 1945, and seeing the flag raised on Mount Suribachi through his binoculars.[34]

At the end of 1946, the postwar impact was even more pronounced. The total enrollment in the fall 1946 term had increased to 15,564 undergraduates, 13,382 men and 2,182 women. Clearly the percentage of women had significantly decreased even as the actual number increased. Of the 13,382 men, 10,586 were veterans.[35] In a 1947 survey the Veterans Administration reported that there were almost 1,300 disabled veterans studying pharmacy.[36]

CREDIT FOR MILITARY EXPERIENCE

The issue of college credit for military experience was raised as early as 1944. Pharmacy leaders in state boards and the colleges were concerned that men trained in the military short courses would demand that they be given a pharmacy license on the basis of their military experiences. After all, the logic went, if these men were competent enough to provide pharmacy services in the military they were also competent enough to provide them in civilian life. There was

TABLE 8.1. Winter Term 1945-1946 Enrollment in College of Pharmacy

Classes	Men 4-F	Men under 18	Selective Service— eligible men	Male veterans	Female veterans	Total men enrolled	Total women enrolled	Total in class
Freshmen	308	310	401	2,437	16	3,460	763	4,223
Sopho- mores	235	29	108	722	4	1,151	554	1,705
Juniors	187	5	33	418	2	689	360	1,049
Seniors	148	0	24	218	1	447	239	686
Special	10	0	1	100	1	157	48	205
Graduate	32	0	3	50	2	116	20	136
Totals	920	344	570	3,945	26	6,020		

Note: All honorably discharged veterans were eligible for the GI Bill. No school- or state-specific tally of those going to school on the GI Bill has been located.

also the realization that the returning serviceman was a member of a "powerful organization backed to the limit by public opinion."[37]

In late 1944 the American Association of Colleges of Pharmacy and National Association of Boards of Pharmacy reviewed the issue, taking special note of the 250 courses offered by the Armed Forces Institute to Army and Navy personnel. The institute listed pharmacy in the subjects to be offered but no specific courses, which made it unlikely that anyone could take a pharmacy course for college credit. The commandant recommended that no college credit be given for experience in pharmaceutical service but suggested that the boards of pharmacy consider such experience in lieu of part of the practical experience requirement.[38]

The American Council on Pharmaceutical Education also appointed a committee to review the issue of granting educational credits for military experience. The committee surveyed a small group of universities to determine what policies were already in place. The ACPE committee recommended that the colleges provide no educational credit for military pharmacy experience and that credit, if given, should be by the boards in lieu of part of the practical experience. Any credit for practice experience was a state board issue which meant that practice experience in the military could be allowed. Credit could be allowed for military experiences such as basic training in place of physical education or hygiene requirements. Finally, college credits should be allowed only for equivalent courses on a degree level; and it would be important to test for content rather than simply accept the number of hours taken.[39]

Robert Fischelis served on both of the committees considering credit for military service. He summarized his position on the topic in a 1945 editorial, "Give the Veteran His Due," after he became the secretary of the American Pharmaceutical Association. Framing his comments in the context of pharmacists' societal responsibility for public health, he questioned the wisdom of allowing someone to practice pharmacy without the fundamental training that would enable him to practice most effectively in the public interest. Such a gift would be false when the postwar fervor wore off and pharmacists once again competed for positions on the basis of what they knew and could do. Financial hardships were not the barrier they had once been since every veteran had the GI Bill to pay school costs and provide a stipend for living expenses.

> Standards of pharmaceutical education and licensure are not "commodities" to be handed out freely by generous pharmacists or legislatures. They are responsibilities entrusted to the profession which must be jealously guarded and which should be dispensed only with due care for the interests of the people of the United States and the profession which the people rely upon to maintain adequate health care.[40]

Many veterans were unable to apply their military experiences to their postwar education. For example, John Mullins was a P-38 fighter pilot in Europe. Upon his discharge in 1945 his first choice was aeronautical engineering, a popular choice for those with military experience in the Air Force and one that was already overcrowded. After taking some math courses in a junior college he was accepted in 1946 at the Massachusetts College of Pharmacy. The college arranged a part-time job (with no pay) that would provide the necessary drugstore experience to qualify him for admittance. His class, he wrote, was

> 90% veterans and out of the 150 there were six girls. We treated the non-veterans and girls like kid brothers and sisters. The rest of us were there for a purpose, we attended class and went from school to work in one of the local pharmacies. It was very much a no-nonsense, nose to the grindstone four years. We were there for an education and there was little room for extracurricular activity.[41]

CIVIL SERVICE

On October 24, 1945, the Civil Service Commission released Position Announcement 404 for pharmacists with war service. The requirements for positions included three years of technical experience, a bachelor's degree in pharmacy, or a combination of the two.[42] The duration of the appointment was limited to six months after the legal termination of the war. The fact that individuals would be hired for government positions in spite of the fact that they could not qualify for registration in forty-five of the forty-eight states created immediate reactions from both the American Pharmaceutical Association and NARD. Fischelis wired a protest of the announcement to both President Truman and the president of the Civil Service Commission, Harry B. Mitchell, and copied the materials to state boards, associations, and colleges.[43]

Fischelis and Mitchell exchanged a series of letters for the rest of 1945. Mitchell took the position that the Civil Service was merely carrying out the intent of Congress as expressed in the Veterans' Preference Act of 1944 and that there was no guarantee that individuals without a BS degree could pass the Civil Service exam. In particular Mitchell took the position that Civil Service was proscribed from establishing minimum educational requirements for scientific or technical positions which can be performed by individuals without the degree requirements. He argued that since more than half of all pharmacists were practicing legally without a BS degree, there was not sufficient evidence to require a college education.[44]

Fischelis' response was that Mitchell misunderstood the fact that state boards had been insisting on a college degree as a prerequisite for licensure since 1905; that no college accepted students for less than a three-year course after 1925; and that the four-year BS curriculum had become mandatory in 1932. The underlying concern of organized pharmacy was that the "experience-only" criteria would be used by cram school operators to encourage those with military experience to take the course in the hope of gaining a job with the federal government.[45]

The issue was finally settled on January 3, 1946, with the passage of HR 4717, an enactment to establish a Department of Medicine and Surgery in the Veterans Administration. The law provided for the appointment of a chief pharmacist who was to be the principal advisor to the chief medical director. As part of the law, qualifications were established for pharmacists in the VA under Civil Service. The qualifications included U.S. citizenship, having a BS degree or its equivalent from an approved college of pharmacy, and being a registered pharmacist.[46] On January 11, 1946, Harry B. Mitchell wrote to Robert Fischelis announcing that the examinations under Civil Service Announcement 404 were canceled due to the passage of HR 4717.[47]

While it seemed that the problem was solved, another was created, as some pharmacists without a BS complained that they were excluded from Civil Service and Veterans Administration or were being relegated to paraprofessional positions.

The first chief pharmacist of the Veterans Administration was William Paul Briggs, a former dean of the George Washington School of Pharmacy and an officer in the Navy during the war. At the end of 1947 he reviewed the status of the Veterans Administration and pharmacy's place in it. He noted that there were currently 3 million men and women receiving VA pharmaceutical services with a potential of 18 million. The problems being treated were the result of trauma from combat as well as diseases contracted in all parts of the world. Over 200 pharmacies were staffed by more than 350 VA pharmacists. In addition to providing ward supplies in the hospital, over 4 million prescriptions had been filled the previous year.[48]

PHARMACY CORPS

By 1945 the APhA Steering Committee on the Status of Pharmacists in the Government Service and other pharmacy leaders were becoming vocal about what was perceived as the poor faith of the Army's surgeon general in implementing the Pharmacy Corps Bill. Arthur Einbeck, the chair of the committee and a retired Army officer, published articles in the professional press reviewing the status of pharmacists in the Army. He noted that those pharmacists who had gained commissions as pharmacists in 1936 had been scattered through the service to the point where they could no longer be identified.[49] Aggravating the situation was the War Department's Circular 392 of December 29, 1945, which waived the educational requirements for the Pharmacy Corps and solicited applications from optometry, clinical psychology, and other technical fields for commissions in the Pharmacy Corps. George Frates, the NARD Washington representative, wrote, in a furious vein, that the "Brass Hats" had given the Pharmacy Corps the "Brush Off." [50]

On February 15, 1946, Surgeon General Kirk and some of his staff members, including pharmacists Major Bernard Aabel and Major Frank L. McCarthy, met with pharmacy leaders at the APhA headquarters. Kirk explained his plan to form a Medical Service Corps that would include the Sanitary Corps, the Medical Administrative Corps, and the Pharmacy Corps. The plan included the establishment of a pharmacist officer to serve in the office of the surgeon general to advise him on all pharmacy matters and direct the pharmaceutical services of the Medical Department. The initial response of pharmacy leaders was negative; the committee promised to oppose the new corps since it meant the abolishment of the Pharmacy Corps.[51] Kirk named Aabel his assistant for pharmacy affairs with the assignment to act as a liaison between his office and pharmacy leadership.[52] Aabel was an excellent choice for the assignment. A graduate of the University of Minnesota College of Pharmacy in 1932, he had practiced in retail pharmacy until 1940. Aabel was assigned as the intelligence and liaison officer for the 68th Medical Group when he landed on Omaha Beach in 1944 and was later wounded. After the war he was assigned to the Surgeons General's staff.*

In June 1946 pharmacy leadership provided General Kirk with a "blue print" of the role that pharmacy could play in the Army. The "blue print" proposed the minimum educational requirements for Army pharmacists. In addition, it provided the vision for the functions and responsibilities of the Pharmacy Corps, including the "responsibility for medical supply tables, preparation of standards, procurement, command functions, responsibility for training of enlisted men, teaching in Medical Field Service Schools, compounding and dispensing of medicines, hospital functions, combat organizations, medical and general laboratory."[53] The proposal was received positively since Kirk felt that it largely matched his goal of improving pharmacy services in the Army. On July 5 Kirk announced that he would seek legislation establishing a new Medical Service Corps. The Pharmacy Corps would become a section of that new organization and be charged with "the purchase, storage, examination, shipment, and standardization of drugs and medical supplies."[54] Eventually, pharmacy agreed to support the legislation proposed by Surgeon General Kirk with the understanding that pharmacy would

---

*Aabel was assigned as a military attaché in Finland in 1948. In 1955 he became the third chief of the Medical Service Corps. Ginn, R.V.N. (1977). *The History of the U.S. Army Medical Service Corps Office of the Surgeon General and the Center of Military History.* Washington, DC: U.S. Army, p. 481.

be an integral part of the new corps. This was facilitated by the appointment of James H. Kidder, dean of the Fordham University College of Pharmacy, as a consultant to the surgeon general. Kidder was also a physician who served in Europe and was a friend of many of the surgeon general's staff.[55] Othmar Goriup was named the first commander of the newly formed Medical Service Corps. Goriup, a 1929 graduate of the University of Pittsburgh College of Pharmacy, practiced in a retail pharmacy before entering active service in 1941. Assigned to the Army Air Corps, he served as the chief of the Supply and Operations Division in the headquarters of the Air Transport Command.[56]

THE NAVY

Matters went somewhat differently in the Navy. When the Pharmacy Corps legislation was passed in 1943 the Committee on the Status of Pharmacists in Government Service had worked to create a similar organization in the Navy. This was never effected, due in large part to the positive relationship Navy Surgeon General Ross McIntire and his predecessors had maintained with pharmacy. On August 5, 1944, a commitment was made to APhA to seek legislation for a commissioned hospital corps which would have pharmacists as an integral part. The commitment proposed to "assign as many pharmacy officers on duty in connection with the specifications, purchase, storage, inspection, distribution, and dispensing of drugs and medical supplies as may be utilized efficiently in these capacities."[57] By May 6, 1946, there was agreement that the Navy would discontinue the use of pharmacist mate as a rank and that 20 percent of the commissioned officers in the new Commissioned Hospital Corps would be graduates of colleges accredited by the American Council on Pharmaceutical Education.[58]

THE MEDICAL SERVICE CORPS

In February 1947 house hearings were held on HR 1982 "to establish a permanent Medical Service Corps in the Medical Department of the Regular Army." Margaret Chase Smith, chair of the House

Committee on Armed Services, decided to include HR 1361 "to establish commissioned medical administrators in the Navy's Hospital Corps" and HR 1603 "to establish a Navy Medical Associated Sciences Corps" in the hearings. On August 4, 1947, Congress passed the Army-Navy Medical Services Corps Act. The Pharmacy Corps was gone, but with its demise commissioned status was gained for pharmacists to practice pharmacy in the Army and Navy. That licensed pharmacists had the responsibility to provide pharmaceutical services in the military had become the law of the land.

CONCLUSION

In a note at the beginning of *"The Good War,"* Studs Terkel noted the incongruity of the adjective and the noun in the explanation for the use of the quotes in the title.[59] In *Days of Sadness, Years of Triumph: The American People, 1939-1945,* Geoffrey Perrett uses the sobriquet the "perfect war."[60] In spite of the obvious incongruity, the war was an important and mostly positive episode for pharmacy.

Pharmacy practice during the war was economically strong. If net profits and the low number of stores that closed due to financial failure are any measure, retail pharmacy enjoyed economic success. Store hours were shorter, relieving the pharmacist and his staff from grueling sixteen hour days, seven days a week. Many consumer products were either not available or rationed during the war. This forced a return to the prescription counter and health care products that were the hallmark of the health profession.

Educational standards were upheld in spite of tremendous pressures to abandon them. The bachelor's degree was maintained as the educational entry to the profession. While the four-year program was squeezed into thirty-six months, the basic criteria for licensure was maintained. Licensure standards of experiential training were scrutinized as never before; at stake was the acceptance of national standards that would allow for the freedom of movement through reciprocity in the postwar world.

After an adversarial relationship that continued forty-nine years and through the terms of office of ten surgeons generals, the Army recognized pharmacy as a health profession. Although the Pharmacy

Corps did not exist as a separate organization for long, the foundation for commissioning pharmacists to practice pharmacy in the military was established.

The GI Bill brought both prosperity and frustration to the colleges as veterans returned from the military service. People who could never dream of going to college before the war were not only dreaming of it, they were doing it. The influx of mature and experienced men and women challenged what was being taught and how it was being taught. The veterans wanted reality and practicality in their education, and they had the maturity to expect and demand it.

Changes in practice accelerated in the poswar period; compounding had been in a steady decline even before the war. New products and technologies developed during the war burst into the local drugstores. The era of the miracle drugs started, with penicillin, streptomycin, blood products, and other advances. More prescriptions were being written and filled; the American public had new expectations for health and health care.

A new generation of pharmacy leaders emerged from their experiences during the war, both civilian and military. New professional organizations such as the American Society of Hospital Pharmacists and the American College of Apothecaries, which had been formed during the war, gained acceptance and leaders. More women entered the profession not only to fill the schools during the war but as an ongoing part of the profession.

Perrett concluded:

> The war experience is as close as this country has ever come to living the American Dream. Vague through that phrase is, if it means anything at all, it is that America has something for everybody. A wildly heterogeneous nation was more completely united in purpose and spirit than at any time in its history. That in itself was a rich emotional experience. It gave everyone a vital sense of community . . . the triumph over foreign enemies was a lesser victory than the war generation's victory over its own history. They—the living embodiment of the country's history—faced the test of mastering a historic challenge—and succeeded. Old myths and institutions were tested, new ones were created.[61]

Chapter 9

Postscript

There has never been a census of the pharmacists and pharmacy students who served in the military during World War II. Estimates of pharmacists in the American Armed Forces ranged from 10,000 to 14,000, but these never included a basis for the numbers cited.* There were no national estimates of the number of students who served, but, given the enrollment decline, thousands would be a reasonable estimate.

As part of my research I contacted every state association, board of pharmacy, and college of pharmacy of the period asking for information about pharmacists and students. Few had records they remembered or could find, but many published a notice of my search in their journals, newsletters, and bulletins. While this approach elicited responses from 335 individuals (see Appendix IV), it did not answer the questions of how many served and who they were.

I spent a great deal of time scanning state, regional, and national journals of the period. I found that these publications frequently contained the names of individuals in the military and sometimes snippets of information about colleges attended, years of graduation, promotions, wounds, and deaths. The information from these sources was inconsistent and incomplete. Some publications listed names of men and women in the service without identifying the branch. Sometimes a similar or same name appeared in different states with no evidence that they referred to the same individual. A similar problem

---

*The estimates of the numbers who served are as inconsistent as the estimates of the number of pharmacists were at the beginning of the war. George A. Moulton estimated that 10,000 registered pharmacists served in the military. Moulton, George A. (1945). "A Report on Wartime Pharmacy." *The Apothecary,* 57(July):11, 14, 16, 18. Charles Gilson, a member of the NARD executive committee, estimated that 14,000 served. Gilson, Charles (1945). "A Retail Druggist Looks at Postwar Pharmacy." *NARD Journal,* 67(November 19):2015, 2060, 2062.

arose when an individual was identified in one place by initials and in another by a nickname or full name.

In spite of the inconsistencies, I decided to build a database with the names and the information that I was able to find from any source. While there were problems, they were not significant enough to abandon the effort. Use of the information in the database, however, is always accompanied by the caveat that there are possible errors.

The database includes pharmacists, pharmacy students, and those who returned from the military and attended pharmacy school on the GI Bill. Where known, the branch of service (Army, Navy, Army Air Force, Marines, Coast Guard, and Merchant Marines) and whether the individual was commissioned is included. The state of residence given by the source is also included. In the case of the national and regional journals this information was frequently not given and, therefore, is not included in the database. Where possible, information on the pharmacy school and year of graduation is listed. Also noted are those who were killed in action, died in the service, or were wounded in action. Each name has at least one source reference.

As of December 31, 2003, the database contained 10,826 names of individuals who served in the Armed Forces during World War II. The branch of service is identified for 6,293 individuals (58 percent) and had the following distribution: 2,902 served in the Army (46 percent of those of known service branch); 2,489 in the Navy (40 percent); 572 in the Army Air Force (9 percent); 125 in the Marines (2 percent); 66 in the Coast Guard (1 percent); and 50 in the Merchant Marines (less than 1 percent). The remaining 1 percent were women who served in the military; 25 in the WAAC (later WAC), 40 in the WAVES, and 5 in the SPARS. It may be more accurate to consider the Army and Army Air Forces as one unit and the Navy and Marines as another, since medical care was provided by the Army and by Navy for the other two branches. Men in the Army Air Force were frequently listed as being in the Army, those in the Marines as in the Navy.

While few individuals were commissioned to serve as pharmacists, many were commissioned for other assignments. Of the total database, 16 percent (1,783 of 10,765) were commissioned; 13 percent of these (206) were pharmacy students who left their education to serve.

A large number of pharmacy students interrupted their studies to serve in the military; 1,132 are listed in the database. Many of these students returned to pharmacy school on the GI Bill after the war. The database also contains the names of many who began their pharmacy education after the war on the GI Bill. The database contains 562 individuals, both returning and new students, using the GI Bill.

A number of men died during their military service. Most of these men were killed overseas, in action. One hundred thirty-one (1.2 percent of all serving in the military) are known (see Appendix VI).

The database may be accessed at the American Institute of the History of Pharmacy Web site (www.aihp.org). The database will be updated several times a year to include new names and information. Readers are requested to send corrections and additions to the author at dbworthen@fuse.net or to the institute.

Appendix I

Colleges and Schools of Pharmacy, 1944

State	College	Dean or Director
AL	Howard College, Birmingham (renamed Samford in 1965)	Leon W. Richards
	Alabama Polytechnic Institute (renamed Auburn in 1960)	Lynn S. Blake
CA	University of Southern California	A. G. Hall
	University of California	Troy C. Daniels
CO	University of Colorado	David W. O'Day
CT	University of Connecticut	H. S. Johnson
DC	George Washington University (discontinued 1964)	Charles W. Blivin
	Howard University	Chauncey I. Cooper
FL	University of Florida	P. A. Foote
GA	University of Georgia	Robert C. Wilson
	Southern College of Pharmacy (merged with Mercer in 1959)	R. C. Hood
ID	University of Idaho, Southern Branch	E. O. Leonard
IL	University of Illinois	Earl R. Serles
IN	Purdue University	Glenn L. Jenkins
	Indianapolis College of Pharmacy (merged with Butler in 1945)	Edward H. Niles
IA	State University of Iowa	R. A Kuever
	Drake University	George E. Crossen
KS	University of Kansas	J. A. Reese
KY	Louisville College of Pharmacy (merged with the University of Kentucky in 1947)	G. L. Curry

State	College	Dean or Director
LA	Loyola University (discontinued in 1964)	John F. McCloskey
	Xavier University	Lawrence L. Ferring
MD	University of Maryland	Andrew G. DuMez
MA	Massachusetts College of Pharmacy	H. C. Newton
	Boston College of Pharmacy (renamed New England College of Pharmacy in 1949, became part of Northeastern in 1962)	
MI	Ferris Institute	Howard Hopkins
	Detroit Institute of Technology (merged with Wayne State in 1957)	Esten P. Stout
	University of Michigan	Howard B. Lewis
	Wayne University	Roland T. Lakey
	Grand Rapids University (never accredited; closed in 1945)	
MN	University of Minnesota	Charles H. Rogers
MS	University of Mississippi	Elmer L. Hammond
MO	St. Louis College of Pharmacy	A. F. Schlichting
	Kansas City University	T. T. Dittrich
MT	University of Montana	C. E. Mollett
NE	Creighton University	William A. Jarrett
	University of Nebraska	Rufus A. Lyman
NJ	Rutgers University	Ernest Little
NY	Fordham University (discontinued in 1975)	Charles J. Deane
	Albany College of Pharmacy	Frances J. O'Brien
	St. John's University	John L. Dandreau
	Columbia University (discontinued in 1976)	C. W. Ballard
	Brooklyn College of Pharmacy (Long Island University)	Hugo H. Schaefer
	University of Buffalo	A. B. Lemon
NC	University of North Carolina	J. G. Beard
ND	North Dakota Agricultural College	W. F. Sudro
OH	Ohio Northern University	R. H. Raabe

State	College	Dean or Director
	Western Reserve University (discontinued 1949)	F. J. Bacon
	University of Toledo	Bess G. Emch
	Ohio State University	Bernard V. Christensen
	Cincinnati College of Pharmacy (merged with the University of Cincinnati in 1954)	L. J. Klotz
OK	University of Oklahoma	D. B. R. Johnson
OR	Oregon State University	Adolph Ziefle
PA	Philadelphia College of Pharmacy and Science	Ivor Griffith
	Temple University	H. Evert Kendig
	University of Pittsburgh	C. Leonard O'Connell
	Duquesne University	Hugh C. Muldoon
RI	Rhode Island College of Pharmacy and Allied Science (merged with the University of Rhode Island in 1957)	W. Henry Rivard
SC	Medical College of South Carolina	William A. Prout
	University of South Carolina	E. T. Motley
SD	South Dakota State College	F. J. LeBlanc
TN	University of Tennessee	R. L. Crowe
TX	University of Texas	W. F. Gidley
VA	Medical College of Virginia	W. F. Rudd
WA	University of Washington	Forest J. Goodrich
	State College of Washington	P. H. Dirstine
WV	University of West Virginia	J. Lester Hayman
WI	University of Wisconsin	Arthur H. Uhl

Appendix II
State Selective Service Pharmacy Advisory Committees

State	Advisory Committee Members*	
AL	E. W. Gibbs (chair)	C.T. Burkart
	Lehman Alley	Paul Molyneux
	Maury McWilliams	L.S. Blake
	Thelma Morris Colburn	
AR	L. K. Snodgrass (chair)	J. B. Ketcham
	C. R. Counts	Fred Veazey
	Irl Brite	
AZ	Newell Stewart (chair)	Arthur Lee Phelps
	Carroll M. Wood	Charles M. Nielson
	H. E. Laird	
CA	Roy S. Warnack (chair?)	Walter B. Stoner
	Walter Gnerich	A. J. Afleck
	John S. Ramsay	Alvah G. Hall
	Henry Kane	C. W. Peters
	Troy C. Daniels	Willard G. Smith
CT	Hugh Beirne (chair)	Robert Benham
	Nicholas Feeney	William Dunphy
	Sidney Curran	Dwight G. Stoughton
	Robert O. Judson	Samuel S. McCulley
DC	Harold C. Kinner (chair)	Morris G. Goldstein
	W. H. Whittlesey	Clayton Aldrich
	David Maxwell	

*A set of questionnaires providing the identities of the state advisory boards is located in the American Pharmaceutical Association Archives.

State	Advisory Committee Members	
DE	Albert Bunin (chair)	John O. Bosley
	George W. Brittingham	Walter E. Brown
	Ruben Kaufman	George W. Rhodes
	Hughett K. McDaniel	
FL	R. Q. Richards	Don S. Evans
	P. A. Foote	Dave Weaver
	A. B. Ware	E. J. Pierce
GA	Z. O. Moore (chair)	J. L. Hawk
	R. L. Brewer	M. D. Hodges
	R. M. Mitchell	
IA	Otto A. Bjornstad (chair)	J. F. Rabe
	R. A. Kuever	M. F. Coontz
	George E. Crossen	
ID	E. O. Leonard (chair)	J. P. Halliwell
	A. A. Walker	
IL	Thomas B. Bolger (chair)	Jo S. Stotlar
	H. E. Strickrod	A. L. Starshak
	E. R. Serles	Thomas J. Vratney
	A. Lee Adams	Joseph R. Oberman
	Joseph Allegretti	
IN	E. H. Niles (chair)	G. L. Jenkins
	Edgar A. O'Harrow	B. M. Keene Sr.
	Chris Iverson	H. V. Darnell
KS	Gene Cook (chair)	Frank Dale
	W. F. Sprague	Blaine Miller
	J. Allen Reese	Elmer Slaybaugh
KY	E. M. Josey (chair)	Marion Hardestty
	A. P. Markendorf	Stanley Ulrey
	Charles H. Tye	Robert H. Wyatt
	J. E. Croley	Cyril Duncan
MD	L. M. Kantner (chair)	Andrew G. DuMez
	Simon Solomon	T. Ellsworth Ragland

State	Advisory Committee Members	
	Harry S. Harrison	Melville Strasburger
MI	J. L. Brown (chair)	F. H. Taft
	Howard B. Lewis	Ben Bialk
	Fred Baxter	Howard Curtis
	Leslie A. Wikel	Otis F. Cook
MN	Charles H. Rogers (chair)	Frank W. Moudry
	Sam Lavine	J. E. Treat
	W. C. Kregel	Porter Remington
	Jesse B. Slocum	R. A. Callender
	Angus H. Taylor	
MO	J. Doyle Norris (chair)	M. C. McGreevy
	Keith L. Karnes	Leonard J. Dueker
	G. D. Tenkhoff	Ted D. Willard
	O. R. Sutton	
MS	Charles E. Wilson (chair)	M. Kelly Patterson
	N. S. Fox	H. H. Jones
	D. B. Sharron	Elmer L. Hammond
	Lew Wallace	
ND	Burt Finney (chair)	Homer L. Hill
	Albert Doerr	W. F. Sudro
	Gus Samuelson	P. H. Costello
	Simon L. Mark	C. B. Hay
NE	M. D. Gulley	Charles H. Sprague
	William A. Jarrett	Oscar E. Geist
	William G. Clayton	H. L. Bellamy
	Louis J. Stewaart	Theo H. McCosh
NH	Rodney A. Griffin (chair)	George A. Moulton
	Percy J. Callaghan	John R. Kelly
	Fred W. Coleman	John A. Greenway
	John H. Mathes	
NJ	Robert J. Fischelis (chair)	Emil P. Martini
	Charles Schamach	Adolph V. Palumbo

State	Advisory Committee Members	
	Percy H. Jackson	Ernest Little
	John J. Debus	Harry B. Reibel
NY	A. B. Lemon (chair)	Arthur Wardle
	Frank Emma	Harry Honikel
	Henry Wildhack	Charles Ballard
	Robert R. Gerstner	Marty H. Sasmor
	Nicholas S. Gesoalde	J. J. Goldberg
OH	M. N. Ford (chair)	B. V. Christensen
	V. L. Keys	P. R. Barnes
	L. W. Funk	
OK	Cal Arnold (chair)	W. C. Alston
	W. B. Irby	W. R. Franklin
	Roger Jones	W. D. Patterson
	Albert Eaton	C. F. Miles
OR	Adolph Ziefle	Ross Plummer
	Earl Gunther	Edgar Stipe
	W. W. Parsons	
PA	George L. McMillin (chair)	Leon A. Spielman
	Martin Bambrick	W. Thomas Senseman Jr.
	Chauncey E. Rickard	
SC	S. B. Michell (chair)	W. L. Califf
	J. D. Ashmore	E. B. Bridgers
	J. M. Plaxco	
SD	Floyd J. LeBlanc (chair)	Floyd M. Cornwell
	Carl Anderson	M. C. Beckers
	T. E. Hulstead	Bliss C. Wilson
	Charles Locke	Thomas Haggar
	Frank E. Kelly	
TN	Tom C. Sharp (chair)	P. P. Vance
	R. L. Crowe	H. J. Berryhill
	R. B. Creech	
TX	Walter Cousins Jr. (chair)	W. F. Gidley

State	Advisory Committee Members	
	Villa Saunders	Gilbert Hermes
	R. L. Brusenhan	
UT	Sam Hariman (chair)	Earle F. Gardemann
	J. B. Heinz	
VA	A. L. I. Winne (chair)	W. F. Rudd
	W. E. Locke	C. E. Webber
	C. L. Guthrie	
WA	L. D. Bracken (chair)	P. H. Dirstine
	Forest J. Goodrich	R. B. Doane
	H. E. Henderson	
WI	Karl Henrich (chair)	Oscar Haertlein
	Max M. Lemberger	Ernest Druechke
	Oscar Rennebohm	A. H. Uhl
	Jennings Murphy	
WV	J. Lester Hayman (chair)	Roy B. Cook
	H. A. Goodykoontz	Fred C. Allen
	George B. Kenney	
WY	R.D. Dame	H. H. Cordiner
	A. E. Roedel	R. S. Halliwell
	Karl Moedl	

Appendix III

Directory of Pharmacy Organizations and Leaders*

NATIONAL PHARMACY ORGANIZATION PRESIDENTS

	APhA	AACP	NABP	NARD
1939-1940	Andrew G. DuMez	Charles H. Rogers	Patrick H. Costello	Albert Fritz
1940-1941	Charles H. Evans	H. Evert Kendig	S. H. Dretzka	Samuel Watkins
1941-1942	Bernard V. Christensen	Rudolph A. Kuever	Paul Molyneux	Hugh Bierne
1942-1943	Roy Bird Cook	Howard C. Newton	Charles Bohrer	J. Otto Kohl
1943-1944	Ivor Griffith	Forest J. Goodrich	A. Lee Adams	J. Otto Kohl
1944-1945	George A. Moulton	Glenn L. Jenkins	R. D. Dame	J. Otto Kohl
1945-1946	George A. Moulton	Glenn L. Jenkins	R. D. Dame	J. Otto Kohl

NATIONAL ASSOCIATIONS, 1944

Association	Secretary
American Association of Colleges of Pharmacy	Clark T. Eidsmore (from 1942) Zada Mary Cooper (until 1942)
American College of Apothecaries	Charles V. Shelby
American Drug Manufacturer's Association	Carson P. Frailey

*Lists are based on the Pharmaceutical Directory (1944), *Journal of the American Pharmaceutical Association, Practical Pharmacy Edition* 5:187-190.

Association	Secretary
American Institute for the History of Pharmacy	Jennings Murphy
American Pharmaceutical Association	Robert P. Fischelis (from 1945)
	Evander F. Kelly (until 1945)
American Pharmaceutical Manufacturer's Association	C. R. Rohrer
American Society of Hospital Pharmacists	I. T. Reamer
Conference of Pharmaceutical Association Secretaries	Clara B. Miller
Federal Wholesale Druggists Association	Ray C. Schlotterer
National Association of Boards of Pharmacy	Patrick H. Costello
National Association of Retail Druggists	John W. Dargavel
National Wholesale Druggists Association	E. L. Newcomb
Proprietary Association	Charles P. Tyrrell

STATE ASSOCIATIONS, 1944

Association	Secretary
Alabama	Thelma M. Coburn
Arizona	N. W. Stewart
Arkansas	Irl Brite
California	Roy S. Warnack
Colorado	Charles J. Clayton
Connecticut	Alice-Esther Garvin
Delaware	Albert Bunin
District of Columbia	Harold C. Kinner
Florida	R. Q. Richards
Georgia	Russell Rainey
Idaho	James Lynch
Illinois	Joseph J. Shine
Indiana	H. V. Darnell
Iowa	V. H. Tyler
Kansas	Clara B. Miller
Kentucky	E. M. Josey

Louisiana	E. Bicnel
Maine	Louis H. Galluba
Maryland	Melville Strasburger
Massachusetts	James F. Finneran
Michigan	Harold G. Seyffert
Minnesota	J. B. Slocumb
Mississippi	Charles E. Wilson
Montana	J. A. Riedel
Missouri	O. R. Sutton
Nebraska	Cora Mae Briggs/Marthajane Dearth
Nevada	Lester J. Hilp
New Hampshire	George A. Moulton
New Mexico	Mrs. Howard L. Williams
New Jersey	John J. Debus
New York	Nicholas Gesoalde
North Carolina	William J. Smith
North Dakota	W. F. Sudro
Ohio	Victor Keyes
Oklahoma	Elbert R. Weaver
Oregon	Jack Lynch
Pennsylvania	Chauncey E. Rickard
Rhode Island	James Deery
South Carolina	J. M. Plaxco
South Dakota	Bliss Wilson
Tennessee	Tom S. Sharp
Texas	H. C. Burroughs
Utah	Earle F. Gardemann
Vermont	Mabel B. Clifford
Virginia	A. L. I. Winnie
Washington	H. E. Henderson
West Virginia	J. Lester Hayman
Wisconsin	Jennings Murphy
Wyoming	John B. Tripeny

BOARDS OF PHARMACY, 1944

Board	Secretary
Alabama	E. W. Gibbs
Alaska	Elwyn Swetmann
Arizona	N. W. Stewart
Arkansas	C. R. Crouts
California	John Foley
Colorado	Ralph E. Kemp
Connecticut	Hugh P. Beirne
Delaware	John O. Bosley
District of Columbia	Harold C. Kinner
Florida	R. Q. Richards
Georgia	R. C. Coleman
Idaho	James J. Lynch
Illinois	Philip M. Harman
Indiana	Edgar A. O'Harrow
Iowa	John F. Rabe
Kansas	Elmer H. Slaybaugh
Kentucky	E. M. Josey
Louisiana	K. M. Frank
Maine	Victor Hinkley
Maryland	L. M. Kantner
Massachusetts	Frank A. East
Michigan	E. F. Taft
Minnesota	F. W. Moudry
Mississippi	Chester E. Jones
Montana	Emil Schoenholzer
Missouri	W. C. McGreevy
Nebraska	Oscar Humble
Nevada	R. W. Fleming
New Hampshire	Percy J. Callaghan
New Mexico	Troy Caviness
New Jersey	Robert P. Fischelis

Board	Secretary
New York	Leslie Jayne
North Carolina	F. W. Hancock
North Dakota	Homer L. Hill
Ohio	M. N. Ford
Oklahoma	Roy L. Sanford
Oregon	Linn E. Jones
Pennsylvania	Edmund H. Newton
Rhode Island	Joseph J. Cahill
South Carolina	M. W. Davis
South Dakota	Bliss C. Wilson
Tennessee	Robert T. Walker
Texas	W. H. Cousins
Utah	Rena B. Loomis
Vermont	Fred D. Pierce
Virginia	A. L. I. Winnie
Washington	Carlton I. Sears
West Virginia	Roy Bird Cook
Wisconsin	Sylvester H. Dretzka
Wyoming	H. H. Cordiner

PRINCIPAL NATIONAL PUBLICATIONS, 1944

Name	Editor
American Druggist	John W. McPherrin
American Journal of Pharmaceutical Education	Rufus A. Lyman
American Journal of Pharmacy	Linwood F. Tice
American Professional Pharmacist	John N. McDonnell
Drug Topics and Drug Trade News	Robert L. Swain
Journal of the American Pharmaceutical Association, Practical Pharmacy Edition	Glenn Sonnedecker
Journal of the American Pharmaceutical Association, Scientific Edition	Justin L. Powers
NARD Journal	George Bender

Appendix IV

Memories Project Respondents

In 1995, I began collecting the war year memories of pharmacists and pharmacy students. I devised a survey format that pharmacists could use to provide descriptive data on their schooling, branch of the military and rank, and an outline for memories of their service. Many state associations, boards, and colleges published information about the Memories Project.

Individuals contacted me to provide information about themselves. In a number of cases the information was scanty, little more than the name of their college, graduation year, and their branch of service. Others provided more detail of what they did on the home front or in the military. Children and spouses wrote to tell me of the death of their father or husband and provided what information they could.

Three hundred and thirty five individuals contacted me with their memories; 313 were men and twenty-two women. Seventy-eight did not serve in the armed forces during the war. Forty-three were students when they entered the service; seventy-eight went to school on the GI Bill after the war.

What follows is the list of those who shared. Missing information was not provided by the respondents, and a follow-up letter elicited no further information.

Last Name	First Name, Middle Name	Service	Commis-sioned	School	Graduation Year
Aaronson	Malvin Seibert	Navy		Philadelphia College of Pharmacy	1944
Ackerman	Louis A.	Army	yes	Brooklyn	1950
Adams	John F.			Nebraska	1939
Alderson	Leland B.	AAF		Illinois	1934
Allen	Abraham	Navy		Oklahoma	1950
Altschuler	Robert	Army		Brooklyn	1940
Anderson	David	Army		Medical College of Virginia	

Last Name	First Name, Middle Name	Service	Commis- sioned	School	Graduation Year
Archambault	George F.	Public Health		Massachusetts College of Pharmacy	1931
Ash	Lloyd M.	Navy		Medical University of South Carolina	
Atkins	Robert M.	Army	yes	Florida	1940
Baker	Carl C.	Navy		Butler	1940
Barch	George F.	Navy	yes	Duquesne	1939
Bates	Lester M.				1945
Beatty	Maxine E.			Drake	1947
Becker	Anthony P.	Navy		Creighton	1944
Behar	Solomon	Navy		Brooklyn	1943
Behnk	Ernest Edmund	Army		Rutgers	1941
BelCastro	Patrick F.	Army		Duquesne	1942
Belson	J. Joseph	Navy		Massachusetts College of Pharmacy	1947
Bennett	Henry R.			Albany	1931
Benson	George E.	Navy	yes	Washington	1947
Berkowitz	Frank L.	Army		Brooklyn	1937
Berman	Alex	AAF		St Johns	1937
Best	Albert A.	Navy		Rutgers	1944
Biemesderfer	Jo				
Blake	E. K.	Navy			
Bogash	Robert C.	Army		Philadelphia College of Pharmacy	1950
Bohlman	Vilas A.			Wisconsin	1932
Borland	Raymond M. Jr	Army		Temple	1940
Botsfield	Howard E.	Army		Drake	1942
Branch	Isaac			Brooklyn	1945
Brasky	Herbert	Army		Brooklyn	1941
Braucher	Charles L.	Army		Philadelphia College of Pharmacy	1947
Brewer	Harold David	Navy			1951

Last Name	First Name, Middle Name	Service	Commis-sioned	School	Graduation Year
Brittingham	Fread William	Army		Kansas City	1951
Brodsky	Aaron	Coast Guard		Brooklyn	1939
Broidy	Samuel	Army			
Brooks	Carl	AAF	yes	Cincinnati	1949
Bryant	Charles C.			Nebraska	1932
Buchalter	Ted	Navy		Southern California	1934
Buennagel	Charles	Navy		Butler	1943
Cady	Tom				
Caplan	Theodore B.	Army		Philadelphia College of Pharmacy	1943
Caruso	John A. Sr.	Army		Columbia	1941
Cernosek	Henrietta			Dansforth, Texas	1934
Cianciolo	James A.	Navy	yes	Cincinnati	1947
Clark	Harry E.	Navy		Albany	1949
Clayton	Max W.	Navy		Ohio State	1939
Cohen	Charles	Navy		Brooklyn	1943
Coker	Samuel T.	AAF		Auburn	1951
Craddock	Edmund Jr.	AAF			
Craddock	James Spear	Army			
Cranswick	Harold	Navy			
Cromly	Charles L.	Navy		Toledo	1940
Crone	K.	Army	yes	Buffalo	1937
Crowe	John S.	Army		Albany	1937
Crozier	Gerald I.	AAF		Duquesne	1951
Cunzeman	John L. Jr.	AAF	yes	Maryland	1950
Daskal	Milton	Army		Brooklyn	1940
Datz	Philip	Navy		Brooklyn	1935
De Clemente	August J.	Army			
Dickinson	Victoria D.			Nebraska	1946
Dolezal	Virginia K.			Kansas	1940

Last Name	First Name, Middle Name	Service	Commis- sioned	School	Graduation Year
DrisCollege	Virginia Ann			Creighton	1945
Drucker	Ed			Minnesota	1941
Druschke	Harold A.			Wisconsin	1930
Dudek	Alfred	Army		Ohio Northern	1952
Eberts	Howard H.			Ohio State	1936
Eden	James S.	Army		Ohio Northern	1942
Ehlke	Edmund E.			Washington	1939
Ellinger	James L.	Navy		Washington	1943
Elsener	August L.	Army		Cincinnati	1939
Endow	Edward	Army		University of California SF	1939
Failla	Joseph S.			Loyola	1936
Fannella	Joe	Marines		Fordham	
Ferguson	Dwight L.	Navy		Florida	1938
Fleischer	Leonard T.			Nebraska	1936
Fogel	Mandel (Max)	Merchant Marine		Columbia	1939
Frament	Paul Stanley	Navy		Albany	1941
France	W. G.	Coast Guard		South Dakota	1937
Frankhauser	Willis S.	Army		Kansas	1942
Freed	Patti L.			Butler	1945
Fyman	Lawrence	AAF		Brooklyn	1939
Gadol	Ellis	Navy	yes	Philadelphia College of Pharmacy	1940
Gaffron	Edwin O.	Navy		St Louis College of Pharmacy	1939
Galloway	Roger	AAF		Drake	1940
Gamm	Henry	AAF		South Carolina	1939
Garrett	Marvin Lynn	Navy		Mississippi	1949
Gellman	Paul			George Washington	1939
Gian	Vincent A.	Army		Fordham	1952

Last Name	First Name, Middle Name	Service	Commis- sioned	School	Graduation Year
Gibson	Melvin	Army	yes	Nebraska	1942
Gibson	Robert D.	Navy		Nebraska	
Glover	Douglas			Maryland	
Goodman	Seymour F.				
Goodrich	Thomas E. Jr.	AAF	yes	Texas	1942
Goody-koontz	Harry A. Jr	Army		West Virginia	1948
Goorley	John T.	Army	yes	Ohio State	1930
Gorin	Irving	AAF			
Gosselin	Raymond	Navy	yes	Massachusetts College of Pharmacy	1943
Granberg	Charles Boyd	Army		South Dakota	1942
Green	Stanley	Navy		Brooklyn	1944
Grider	George W.	Army	yes	Kentucky	
Griffenhagen	George Bernard	Army		Southern California	1949
Griffin	Thomas Edison	Army	yes	Minnesota	1940
Griffin	W. L.	Navy		South Carolina	
Guerra	Fernando			Texas	1933
Gunnoe	Honnie B. Jr	AAF		West Virginia	1948
Hagel	Bette (Wefso)			Nebraska	1945
Hagen	John Percy	Navy	yes	North Dakota	1939
Hammerness	Francis C.	Army		Montana	1947
Hanson	Robert R.	Army		Idaho	1947
Hardwick	Marion Joe	Navy		West Virginia	1948
Hargreaves	Richard			Edinburgh	1939
Harris	Lewis E.			Nebraska	1932
Hart	Albert Henry Jr.	Navy		Michigan	1942
Hartlaub	Gregory S.	Army	yes	Cincinnati	1942
Hayashi	George	Army		Michigan	1952
Hazuka	James Edward			Creighton	1944
Hickman	Martha Louise			West Virginia	1948
Higby	Warren J.	Navy		Wayne	1942

Last Name	First Name, Middle Name	Service	Commis-sioned	School	Graduation Year
Holland	Thomas Marshall Jr.	Navy		North Carolina	1942
Holmes	Burton J.	Navy	yes	Minnesota	1940
Horrell	Robert McC.	AAF		West Virginia	1949
Horton	George A.	Army		Brooklyn	1943
Hulsker	Edwin Fay				
Hunter	J. Fred	Army		Southern	1943
Inashima	O. James	Army		Idaho	1947
Iwamoto	Harry K.			University of California SF	1938
Jacknowitz	Samuel	Army		St Johns	1934
Jackson	Robert L.	Navy		Capitol	1937
Janeway	W. C.	Marines		Texas	1947
Jensen-Norman	H. J. (Herb)			Nebraska	1946
Johnson	James W. III	Navy		Maryland	1949
Johnson	Robert K.	Navy		Wisconsin	1948
Johnson	Virginia Bates			Southern California	1945
Jones	William L.	Navy		Mississippi	1950
Jorganson	Virginia Lee			Nebraska	1941
Joscelyn	Alden L.	AAF		Montana	1950
Kaplan	Rich	AAF		Western Reserve	1947
Kasmin	Herman L.	Navy		Brooklyn	1937
Katsin	Charles H.	Navy		Rutgers	1943
Keegan	Budd	Marines		Cincinnati	1947
Keller	Richard J.	Army	yes	Creighton	1940
Kihara	Cisco Jima			Idaho	1930
Kirshner	Myron	AAF		Temple	1943
Kiszkiel	John A.	Navy		Connecticut	1944
Kitabayashi	Sam			University of California SF	1939
Kita	Joseph			University of California SF	1935
Kleven	Azor J. N.	Army		Minnesota	1942
Knox	Guy G. (Pete)	Navy		Idaho	1949

Last Name	First Name, Middle Name	Service	Commis-sioned	School	Graduation Year
Knox	John J.			Purdue	1950
Koerting	Margaret			Nebraska	1931
Kopecky	Frank Henry	Navy	yes	Illinois	1941
Kopecky	Charles	Navy			
Kortz	Louise Schmitz			Minnesota	1936
LaMonica	Manuel D.	Army		Brooklyn	1940
Lamp	C. O.	Navy		Drake	
Lane	Sam	Merchant Marine		Texas	1959
Lantrip	Paul Auxford	Army	yes	Auburn	1934
Lappas	Lewis C.	Navy		Massachusetts College of Pharmacy	1943
Lasslo	Andrew			Czech	
Leonard	Dave	Army	yes	Washington	1939
Lessin	Morris	AAF		Brooklyn	1939
Leuthauser	Norman A.	Army	yes	Nebraska	1940
Levant	Frank A.	Navy	yes	University of California SF	1940
Lischke	John B. Jr.	Army	yes	Butler	1939
Lohr	Joel D.	Marines		Massachusetts College of Pharmacy	1943
Lund	Richard H.	Navy		Drake	1943
Lynch	John R.	Army		Wisconsin	
Mamet	Harvey	Army		Buffalo	1943
Mancusi	Ralph A.	Merchant Marine	yes	Brooklyn	1944
Manley	Emmett Wallace	Army		Purdue	1947
Marchek	Carlyle Steven	Army	yes	Nebraska	1926
Martin	Edgar E. (Jake)			Wichita	1934
Matsuda	Benjamin Sawaji			University of California SF	1935
Mazzola	Nicholas M.	Army	yes	St Louis College of Pharmacy	1942
McBay	Arthur J.	AAF	yes	Massachusetts College of Pharmacy	1942
McCann	Russell F.	Navy		Massachusetts College of Pharmacy	1950

Last Name	First Name, Middle Name	Service	Commis-sioned	School	Graduation Year
McComb	Gene	Navy			
McConnell	Warren E.	Navy	yes	Purdue	1940
McDowell	Norfleet Owen Jr.	Navy		North Carolina	1944
McFarland	Miles F.	Army		Ohio State	1948
McGarvey	Michael M.			Washington State	1941
McHugh	John	Navy		George Washington	1959
McNeill	John Albert	Navy	yes	North Carolina	1940
McNeill	L. J.				
Meiselas	Edwyn	Merchant Marines		Brooklyn	1943
Mendenhall	Ivan L.	Army		Drake	1939
Merrick	Gale D.	Army		Purdue	1950
Meshnick	Murray	Army		Brooklyn	1944
Millard	Kenneth E.	Army	yes	Nebraska	1940
Miller	Jacob W.	Navy		Kentucky	1951
Miller	Dale V.	Navy	yes		
Mishler	John W. Jr	Navy	yes	Creighton	1943
Mitchell	George Clinton	Navy		Cincinnati	1936
Mixon (LaBrune)	Margaret M.	Army		Nebraska	1941
Miya	Midori Sakamoto			Nebraska	1945
Miya	Tom	Army		Nebraska	1947
Money	Jack Presley	Army	yes	Purdue	1941
Mooney	Gene R.	Navy		Cincinnati	1947
Moore	Vernon Robert	Army		Pittsburgh	1949
Moss	Leonard	Army		Brooklyn	1937
Mullins	John	AAF		Massachusetts College of Pharmacy	1950
Mupsak (Mupsik)	Herman M.	Army	yes	Rutgers	1941
Nakamura	Frank			University of California	1938
Neese	Aurel J.	Navy		Texas	1941

Last Name	First Name, Middle Name	Service	Commis-sioned	School	Graduation Year
Nef	Jack V.	Army		Drake	1951
Nekrassoff	Lois Hummel			Tennessee	1945
Ness	Donald J.	Navy		North Dakota	1944
Nettles	Joseph H.	Navy		Tennessee	
Newman	Don Melvin	AAF	yes	Purdue	1947
Noh	Joseph G.	Army	yes	Nebraska	
Okamoto	Shizuo Harold			University of California SF	1936
Olson	Gordon D.	Navy		University of California SF	1940
Olson	Jack	Merchant Marine		Southern California	1953
Ouye	Fred			University of California SF	1933
Palkovacs	Barney B.	Army		Cincinnati	1949
Pannill	William E.	AAF		George Washington	1950
Parker	Martin	Army		Brooklyn	1942
Passmore	Arlie C.	Navy		Southern	1949
Peltz	Abraham			Brooklyn	1938
Peterson	John E.	Navy	yes	Nebraska	1938
Picchioni	Albert L.	Army		Montana	1943
Pickard	Jefferson Franklin	Navy		North Carolina	1943
Pierce	Robert B.			West Virginia	1942
Pietraszek	Ted A.	Navy	yes	Rhode Island	1943
Pindus	Oscar	Army		Brooklyn	1942
Poliakoff	Arthur (Bud)	Army		South Carolina	1937
Powers	David B.	AAF	yes	Columbia	1939
Preston (Pumo)	Andrew Joseph	Navy	yes	St Johns	1943
Quick	Clarence Carl	Marines	yes	Texas	1938
Quintana	Ben A.	Marines		Mississippi	1947
Rack	William	Marines		Washington State	1941
Rahm	George E.	Army		Cincinnati	1942

Last Name	First Name, Middle Name	Service	Commis- sioned	School	Graduation Year
Rainey	Harrison				1951
Rebold	William F.	Army		Cincinnati	1942
Reed	Helen V. (Seitz)			Washington State	1948
Renge	Nabuo	Army		St Louis College of Pharmacy	1944
Robbins	Jacob	Navy		Rutgers	1943
Robbins	Jack	Army	yes	Massachusetts College of Pharmacy	1943
Robinson	Charles W.	Navy	yes	Drake	1940
Rodda	Jack W.	Army	yes	University of California SF	1935
Rogers	Everette M.	Navy	yes	West Virginia	1941
Rubin	Irving	Army	yes	Brooklyn	1936
Rubin	Sheldon L.	Coast Guard		George Washington	1948
Russ	Roger M.	Navy		Philadelphia College of Pharmacy	1937
Rutterer	Paul	AAF		Cincinnati	1951
Safranek	Betty Stehlik			Nebraska	1945
Sakamoto	John	Army		Southern California	1950
Saltzman	Irwin	Army		Columbia	1944
Sanders	Robert T. Jr.	AAF	yes	Purdue	
Saski	Witold			Nebraska	1954
Saunders	Richard F.	Army		Minnesota	1944
Schneider	Maxwell M.	Army	yes	Rutgers	1941
Schneider	Philip C.	Army	yes	Rutgers	1940
Schwartau	Neil W.	Navy	yes	Minnesota	1943
Segel	Marvin	Army	yes	Ohio State	1942
Shapiro	Barnet			Brooklyn	1936
Shell	Robert E.			Ferris	1936
Shimasaki	Fred				

Last Name	First Name, Middle Name	Service	Commissioned	School	Graduation Year
Shimomura	Eddie Kazuo			Washington	
Shuster	Paul E.	Army		Cincinnati	1955
Sideli	Aurelio M.	Army	yes	Brooklyn	1939
Silver	Edward N.	Navy		Connecticut	1949
Silverman	Sidney			Connecticut	1949
Silverman	Saul	Army		St Johns	1949
Skauen	Donald M.			Massachusetts College of Pharmacy	1938
Skibniewski	Xavier F.	Army		Illinois	1940
Slotnick	Pinny	Marines		Massachusetts College of Pharmacy	1949
Smith	Paul F.	AAF	yes	Cincinnati	1950
Smith	Earle Byron	Army	yes	Colorado	1947
Smith	Elizabeth A			Cincinnati	1950
Smith	Grafton				
Smithline	Arthur	Army	yes	Brooklyn	1941
Smithline	Ruth			Brooklyn	1941
Snow	H. Robert Jr.				
Sofer	Robert	Army		Columbia	1938
Somer	Jack	Army		Brooklyn	1942
Sonnedecker	Glenn Allen			Ohio State	1942
Sowell	Wayne L.	Navy		New Mexico	1950
Speier	Eva			Nebraska	1942
Spera	John Thomas	AAF	yes	Philadelphia College of Pharmacy	1949
Spreen	Walter C.	Coast Guard		Cincinnati	1940
Stackhouse	Harry A.	Coast Guard	yes	Creighton	1941
Stamper	Adrian L.	Army		Cincinnati	1945
Stanford	Jim O.				
Stayton	Ernest Norwood			Capital	1930
Steier	Maurice J.	Navy	yes	Creighton	1943

Last Name	First Name, Middle Name	Service	Commis- sioned	School	Graduation Year
Stevens	James B.	Navy	yes	Washington	1948
Stevenson	Ralph S.	AAF		West Virginia	1951
Stevenson	Donald C.	Army	yes	Ohio State	1947
Stewart	Dewey Franklin	Navy		Auburn	
Stock	Fred J.			Purdue	1928
Strauss	George	AAF		Philadelphia College of Pharmacy	1950
Sturgeon	Leonard	AAF		Illinois	
Suzuki	Naoshi	Army		Southern California	1942
Swafford	Wiliam B.	Army		Tennessee	1948
Sweeney	Helen V.	WAVES	yes	Ohio Northern	1941
Takei	Bessie			University of California SF	
Tawshunsky	Ben	AAF		Brooklyn	1938
Taylor	Seymour A.	Merchant Marine		Columbia	1936
Tchon	Irvin R.	AAF		Illinois	1951
Teague	Phil				
Thomas	Heatwole C. (Tommy)	AAF		Tennessee	1950
Timen	Irwin	Army		Brooklyn	1943
Titus	Frank L.	Navy	yes	Southern California	
Tokuda	George			Washington	
Towle	Paula	WAVES	yes	University of California SF	1935
Treese	Lloyd Richard (Dick)	Army		Philadelphia College of Pharmacy	1948
Urbani	Arthur J.	Navy	yes	Pittsburgh	1943
Verme	Dominic A.	Navy		Brooklyn	1950
Vogel	Irving			Brooklyn	1939
Voige	John H. Jr.	Navy	yes	Cincinnati	1943

Last Name	First Name, Middle Name	Service	Commis-sioned	School	Graduation Year
Vranesh	George	Navy			
Walsh	Francis A.	Navy		Creighton	1940
Wanek	Edward F.	Navy		Nebraska	1942
Ware	Bill	Army		Florida	1943
Weaver	Warren E.			Maryland	1942
Weaver	Lawrence C.	AAF	yes	Minnesota	
Weinstein	Raymond L.	Navy		Columbia	1948
Weintraub	Harry	AAF		Florida	1939
Weledniger	Morris	Navy		Brooklyn	1936
Whitford	Bryan H. Jr.	Army		North Carolina	1941
Willingham	Wm R.	Army		Idaho	1949
Wilson	Ray Lee	Navy			
Wolfe	Eddie O.	Coast Guard		George Washington	
Wolfson	Wilfred W.	Army	yes	Florida	1940
Woodyard	James S. (Woody)	Navy		Texas	1942
Yee	Don Moon	Army		University of California SF	1942
Zande	Louis O.				
Ziegenbein	Walter E.	Army	yes	Nebraska	1938
Zonies	Albert	Army		Philadelphia College of Pharmacy	1941
Zuckman	Herman S.	Navy		Columbia	1949
Zugich	John			Illinois	
Zweber	Norbert			North Dakota	

Appendix V

Extracts of the 1943 Medical Department Supply Catalog (Army)

Office of The Surgeon General, Washington

TABLE OF CONTENTS

*Class 1 covers forty pages in the 1942 supply table.

Section III Medical Department Blank Forms
Index

INTRODUCTION

1. **GENERAL.**—The Medical Department Supply Catalog lists the standard items that are procured, stored, and issued by the Medical Department. As indicated by the preceding Table of Contents, this edition is arranged in four parts as follows:

   a. Active Items.—Equipment and supplies are grouped by identifying item numbers under separate classifications according to use. Items appearing in this part of the catalog are those currently purchased and issued by the Medical Department.

   b. Issue While In Stock Items.—These are items for which purchase for the Army has been discontinued, but for which stock remaining from previous purchases will be issued until supply is exhausted. These items are also procured or issued under Lend-Lease. They are classified according to use in the same manner as active items, but have been withdrawn from the numerical location they occupied as active items and constitute the second part of the catalog.

   c. Appendix.—The appendix is composed of three sections as follows:

   Section I lists organizational equipment of the Medical Department and indicates the proper reference source which will provide an itemized breakdown of this equipment.

   Section II lists all kits, chests, cases, etc., procured by the Medical Department, together with the components comprising each assembly.

   Section III lists Medical Department and certain War Department blank forms used for reporting field activities. . . .

4. **ALLOWANCES.**—Based on troop strength, allowances are shown for all expendable items in the catalog except a limited number which are issued only as components of an assembly. Expendable items in Class 8 are designated "As required," and expendable items in other classes used for veterinary purposes may also be requisitioned as required without limitation of the published allowance figures. Allowances for nonexpendable items are not shown in this catalog, since such allowances are governed by the type of installation at which equipment and supplies are to be used.

5. **PRICES.**—The prices shown in this catalog will govern in all cases of charges on payrolls, reports of survey, transfers, inventories, requisitions, and shipping tickets.

6. **REQUISITIONING.**—The following general instructions apply only in the continental United States. . . .

   a. <u>Requisitions for Expendable Items</u>.— . . . Allowances for expendable items are based on troop strength. General hospitals will assume troop strength as the number of beds multiplied by 25. Requirements for expendable items for all organizations and installations at the station will be consolidated and one requisition submitted therefore. Commencing June 1, 1943, the "maximum level" (on hand and on order) expendable items is established for 5 months. Requisitions for expendable items will show on the face thereof, or in the letter of transmittal, troop strength for the current month and the estimated troop strength for next 4 months—a total of 5 months.

  In determining the "maximum level," the projected strength for 5 months will be totaled and this figure, in thousands, will be multiplied by the number appearing in the allowance column of the catalog. Example:

Troop Strength

June	15,000
July	15,000
August	15,000
September	20,000
October	<u>15,000</u>
Total	80,000

Calculation

The allowance for item 10100 Acid, Acetylsalicylic, USP, 5 gr. Tab., is 5.750. Therefore the "maximum level" for this item at this station is 80 times 5.750 or 460.

In applying troop strength; the following instructions will govern:

   1 to 10,000—Nearest 100 figure will be used. Examples: 501 to 549 will be considered 500, while 550 to 599 will be considered 600; 5,501 to 5,549 will be considered 5,500, while 5,550 to 5,599 will be considered 5,800.

   10,000 and above—Nearest 1,000 figure will be used. Example: 13,001 to 13,499 will be considered 13,000, while 13,500 to 13,999 will be considered 14,000.

CLASS 1—DRUGS, CHEMICALS, BIOLOGICAL STAINS

Item	Unit	Unit Price	Allowance per 1,000 Men per Month
Acetone, ACS	pound	0.38	1.2910
Acid, acetylsalicylic, USP	pound	0.96	0.7200
Acid, acetylsalicylic, USP 5 GR tab	1000	1.21	5.7500
Acid, Boric, Ointment USP	4 oz	0.12	1.0000
Acid, Salicylic, USP	¼ lb	0.17	2.1000
Acid, tannic, USP	¼ lb	0.24	0.2922
Alcohol, USP (ethyl)	quart	0.14	0.9450
Alcohol, USP (ethyl)	54 gals	18.09	0.1200
Aloin Compound, pill or tablet	1000	0.52	0.8500
Ammonium chloride, troches, USP	1000	0.52	1.0500
Amyl nitrate, USP, 5 minim, Amp 10	pkg	0.38	0.3732
Antimony and Potassium Tartrate, USP	ounce	0.10	0.0978
Apomorphine Hydrochloride, 1/10 gr hypo tab, USP	20	0.24	0.2132
Arsenic trioxide, USP, 5 gr tab	100	0.15	0.0315
Atabrine tablets, 100 mg	1000	7.50	0.1000
Atropine sulfate, USP ¼ gr Hypo tab	10	0.07	0.0450
Bismuth Subsalicylate, USP, for parenteral injection: (Anti-syphilitic) 60 cc bottle. Sterile	each	1.00	1.2000
Calamine, prepared, NF VI	pound	0.28	1.2375
Capsicum, USP	ounce	0.06	0.0375
Cascara sagrada extract, USP, 2 gr tab	1000	1.60	0.3125
Codeine sulfate, USP ½ gr tab	500	4.45	0.9500
Codeine Sulfate, USP, ½ gr hypo tab	20	0.60	1.2000
Digitalis, tab or capsule, ½ USP XII unit: approx ¾ gr	100	0.35	0.1025
Ephedrine sulfate, NF VI, 1cc amp ¾ gr	dozen	0.60	0.6250
Ergot, 1 cc: equal to 1 cc fl ex ergot, USP	cc	0.04	0.6250
Ether (for anesthesia)	¼ lb	0.10	22.000

Extract belladonna, powdered USP	ounce	0.16	0.1910
Extract Hyoscyamus, powdered, USP	ounce	1.70	0.1336
Fl Ex Cascara Sagrada, aromatic, USP	pint	0.47	1.0500
Foot powder	¼ lb	0.05	46.8000
Glycerin, USP	pound	0.23	1.9445
Glycyrrhiza and opium compound mixture, USP tab	1000	0.54	0.4000
Hydrogen Peroxide, Solution 8 %	pound	0.35	4.8000
Iodine, USP	¼ lb	1.19	1.1250
Ipecac and opium powder, 5 gr tab	500	1.54	0.2500
Jelly, Lubricating: 4 ounce	tube	0.15	2.1000
Liquor carbonis detergens, NF (Solution of coal tar)	pint	2.00	0.1600
Mercurial Ointment, Mild, USP	pound	0.50	1.0833
Mercuric cyanide tablet	100	0.75	0.0625
Mercuric oxide, yellow, ointment, USP	¼ ounce	0.04	5.7500
Mercurous Chloride Ointment, Mild	pound	1.06	2.2000
Morphine sulfate, USP ¼ gr Hypo tab	20	0.14	0.7500
Oil, cod liver, USP	pint	0.27	1.5000
Oil, linseed, USP	gallon	1.25	0.0600
Petrolatum, liquid, heavy, USP	gallon	0.96	1.8750
Petrolatum, liquid, light, USP	pint	0.18	1.4063
Phenolphthalein, USP 2 gr tab	1000	0.62	0.0345
Potassium permanganate, USP	5 lbs	1.35	0.0200
Potassium permanganate, USP 5 gr tabs	100	0.06	0.5209
Procaine hydrochloride, USP, ¾ gr, Hypo tab	20	0.33	1.1340
Quinine sulfate USP 5 gr tab	1000	8.30	1.9700
Sodium bicarbonate and peppermint tab	1000	0.20	1.2500
Sodium bicarbonate, USP 5 gr tab	1000	0.90	0.3976
Sodium salicylate, USP 5 gr tab	1000	0.94	0.6295
Sodium thiosulfate, pea crystals	100 lbs	3.75	0.0760
Strychnine sulfate, USP 1/60 gr Hypo tab	20	0.16	0.2957
Sulfadiazine sodium, USP 5 gm vial: For intravenous use	6	5.00	0.5000

Item	Unit	Unit Price	Allowance per 1,000 Men per Month
Sulfamilamide, USP, 5 gr tab	1000	6.50	0.6000
Sulfanilamide, crystalline, USP, 5 gms in sterile individual double-wrapped envelope: with shaker top	pkg	0.80	2.0000
Sulfapyridine, USP, 7.7 gr tab	1000	5.50	0.3000
Sulfathiazole, USP, 7.7 gr tab	1000	7.00	1.4592
Terpin hydrate, USP	ounce	0.08	2.1000
Tincture opium, camphorated, USP	pint	0.47	1.7333
Whiskey, USP	quart	1.57	1.5252
Zinc oxide ointment, USP	pound	0.28	1.6589

BIOLOGICAL PRODUCTS

Item	Unit	Unit Price	Allowance per 1,000 Men per Month
Antianthrax serum, human, lyophilized 50 cc	vial	5.00	As required
Antitoxin, dysentery, monovalent, Shiga, 20,000 units	vial	4.25	As required
Anthrax serum, 100 cc	vial	1.30	As required
Cholera vaccine, 20 cc	vial	1.50	As required
Gas gangrene antitoxin, polyvalent, without tetanus antitoxin (10,000 each of *Perfringens* and *Vibrion septique* in vial)	vial	6.40	As required
Plague vaccine, 20cc	vial	1.80	As required
Smallpox vaccine, USP 10 capillary tubes in package	pkg	0.50	As required
Tetanus antitoxin, USP 20,000 units	vial	2.90	As required
Tetanus toxoid, plain 30 cc	vial	2.30	As required

Appendix VI

Pharmacists and Pharmacy Students Who Died in Military Service

At least 131 pharmacists and pharmacy students died in the military service; most of them were killed in action. This list is drawn from the source materials that were used in the construction of the database (see Chapter 9) and is probably incomplete. Please send any information on these individuals as well as the names and information on any others to: Dennis B. Worthen, 1723 Old Farm Drive Loveland, OH 45140 or e-mail dbworthen@fuse.net.

Last Name	First Name, Middle Name	Service	School	Comment
Adalman	Melvin S.		Maryland	
Adamczyk	Frank			
Adams	William Howard	Army	Washington State	
Alexander	Charles E.	Navy	Philadelphia College of Pharmacy	July 14, 1944
Allison	Eddie		Washington State	Killed in action (KIA) in the South Pacific
Asal	Jack M.	Army	Montana	Was wounded at Guadalcanal and was being air evacuated to a hospital— plane never arrived
Athas	William P.	Army		Killed by sniper fire at Anzio
Bachelder	Franklin P.	Army	Massachusetts College of Pharmacy	KIA in Germany on February 27, 1945

Last Name	First Name, Middle Name	Service	School	Comment
Ball	Philip Maurice	AAF	Oregon	Killed on a B-17 bombing mission over Germany on January 11, 1944
Banton	Harold L.	Army	Oregon	Died as a result of wounds from the Battle of Leyte
Barvinski	Henry		Temple	
Becker	Casper		Philadelphia College of Pharmacy	
Bellamy	Bob	Marines	Purdue	Bronze Star for meritorious service on Okinawa KIA on May 10, 1935
Berube	Edmund J.		Massachusetts College of Pharmacy	
Black	Raymond M.	Army	Philadelphia College of Pharmacy	July 15, 1943
Blakeslee	Leslie Carlyle	Marines	Connecticut	KIA in the South Pacific
Bookwalter	Lane	AAF	Purdue	
Bradley	Albert	AAF		KIA on December 1, 1944, in air combat over Italy
Brinker	George R.	AAF	Cincinnati	KIA in New Guinea March 12, 1944
Brown	Berwyn E.	Army	Purdue	Killed in Italy January 12, 1944
Brown	Herschel Gordon	Navy	North Carolina	KIA August 2, 1945
Bueltemann	Leonard Weldon		St. Louis College of Pharmacy	

Last Name	First Name, Middle Name	Service	School	Comment
Butel	Gerald A.	Army	Kansas	Lost on December 15, 1944, on a Japanese POW ship
Butler	Alman Byrin Jr.		North Carolina	KIA October 17, 1944
Buza	George E.	Navy	Philadelphia College of Pharmacy	KIA Iwo Jima March 19, 1945
Campanella	Carmelo Ignazio		St. Louis College of Pharmacy	
Carnes	John N.	Marines	Ohio State	December 10, 1943, in the Pacific
Carroll	William J.	Marines	Massachusetts College of Pharmacy	
Casad	Herbert Norwood		St. Louis College of Pharmacy	
Cassidy	W. F.		Columbia	
Chase	Alex		Rutgers	KIA Battle of the Bulge
Cleary	William	Army	Ohio State	KIA in Germany on December 16, 1944
Cole	Jesse Wilson	Army	North Carolina	KIA over Germany November 26, 1944
Cook	Bruce	AAF	Philadelphia College of Pharmacy	KIA in Europe while on unarmed reconnaisance mission
Cooper	L. S.	Navy	Columbia	
Cotterly	Harry R.		Purdue	KIA March 14, 1945
Crabtree	Bynum Griffin	AAF	North Carolina	KIA August 19, 1943, on thirteenth mission over Holland

Last Name	First Name, Middle Name	Service	School	Comment
Craft	Floyd F.	Army	Ohio State	In Germany March 30, 1945
Cudworth	Elmer L.	Army		KIA in France in 1945
Deal	Clarence D.	AAF	St. Louis College of Pharmacy	Shot down over Austria
Docton	Maurice L.	Army	Ohio State	North Africa February 14, 1943
Domino	Joseph	Army	Ohio State	Germany March 19, 1945
Dorsey	Holmes		Kentucky	
Dreyer	Milton	Navy	Iowa	Had been in the Navy but was a civilian on Wake Island when it was captured. KIA October 1943 on Wake
Eisan	Oliver B.	AAF	University of California	Shot down in a B-29 raid over Japan
Farrow	Richard E.	Army	Philadelphia College of Pharmacy	KIA in Belgium on February 7, 1945
Feigin	Mel	AAF	Columbia	
Feingold	Leonard H.	AAF	Massachusetts College of Pharmacy	KIA over Germany
Ferguson	Ralph R.	Army	West Virginia	KIA in Normandy June 14, 1944
Fine	Joseph F.		Maryland	
Forbes	William C.	Army	Philadelphia College of Pharmacy	March, 7, 1943
Forsberg	Harold	Navy	North Dakota	MIA since February 14, 1945
Frament	Paul Stanley	Navy	Albany	KIA in the invasion of Guadalcanal

Last Name	First Name, Middle Name	Service	School	Comment
Freeman	Aubrey	Army	North Dakota	Died while on a Japanese prison ship which was sunk, September 7, 1944
Friedman	William M.	Marines	Philadelphia College of Pharmacy	Participated in the invasions of the Marshalls and Saipan where he was wounded. KIA on Iwo Jima March 20, 1945
Gilbert	Joseph A.	Navy	Purdue	KIA on December 7, 1944, in the Southwest Pacific
Goheen	John R.		Kansas	
Goldberg	Albert		Maryland	
Goldfarb	Albert David	Army	Philadelphia College of Pharmacy	KIA April 1, 1945
Gordon	James S. Jr.	Army	Medical College of Virginia	KIA in the South Pacific on November 12, 1944
Greene	Frank Arthur Jr.	AAF	North Carolina	KIA November 8, 1944, on a dive bombing mission over Metz, Germany
Griffin	John J. Jr.	AAF	Ohio State	Germany October 17, 1943
Harris	Francis G.		Massachusetts College of Pharmacy	
Heath	Marlie Cady	AAF	Michigan	Killed in air action in the South Pacific August 1, 1945
Held	Ralph P.	Army	Ohio State	France February 24, 1945
Horton	George H. Jr.	AAF	Purdue	

Last Name	First Name, Middle Name	Service	School	Comment
Hutchens	Donald Bryce	Army	Oregon	KIA in France
Irvine (Irving)	John Sidney		Tennessee	
Kanetomi	Jero	Army	Washington	KIA in the Vosges Battle
Keitsch	Manfred		Rutgers	KIA Battle of the Bulge
Kerfott	Rolfe	Army	Idaho	KIA in Europe
Kidwell	James		Butler	KIA
Knecht	Robert F.	Army	Cincinnati	KIA when the Germans bombed the hospital base on the Anzio Beachhead February 7, 1944
Knorr	Robert E.	Army	South Dakota	KIA on Cebu Island
Kobiske	Marlyn	AAF	Wisconsin	Killed in Italy June 5, 1944
Koceniak	John J.		Columbia	
Kondo	Henry	Army	University of Southern California	Volunteer with the 442—KIA
LaRue	Richard Van Derlyn	Navy	Philadelphia College of Pharmacy	His ship was torpedoed on November 11, 1942. The rescuing ship was sunk twenty-four hours later and he was killed
Leatherman	Edwin J.	Army	Ohio State	France June 12, 1944
Levine	M. H.	Army	Columbia	
LeWine	Herman E.	Navy	Philadelphia College of Pharmacy	September 11, 1944
London	Sidney (Sol)	Army	Iowa	KIA in France August 8, 1944

Last Name	First Name, Middle Name	Service	School	Comment
Magill	Lloyd Jr.	Army		Captured after the fall of Bataan—KIA on one of the prisoner ships taking POWs to Japan
Malmo	Lee R.	Army	North Dakota	KIA by bomb on Belgian hospital
McMullen	Edward	Army	Connecticut	KIA in Germany on February 9, 1945
Meier	Vernon Arnold	Army	St. Louis College of Pharmacy	KIA September 26, 1944, near the Gothic Line north of Florence, Italy
Michaud	Roland I.	Navy		KIA in South Pacific
Minor	Lee	AAF		KIA in China
Momsen	Leonard		St. Louis College of Pharmacy	
Morris	Ashley D.	Navy	Georgia	KIA November 1942—went down on the cruiser *Atlanta* when it was sunk in action off the Solomon Islands
Nedzinski	Joseph W.		Philadelphia College of Pharmacy	KIA August 1945
Ochs	John			
Parker	Duane Clare	AAF	Michigan	Killed in air action in Europe February 22, 1944
Passwater	Charles		Butler	
Patton	Parke Davis	Navy	Ohio State	Philippines March 4, 1945

Last Name	First Name, Middle Name	Service	School	Comment
Petrick	Marion R.	Army	North Dakota	KIA by a bomb hit on a Belgian hospital
Pfugrath (or Plugrath)	William K.		North Dakota	KIA in the South Pacific on November 22, 1942
Pomponio	Charles	AAF	Massachusetts College of Pharmacy	KIA over Germany
Postle	Ernest N.		Rhode Island	
Powell	Stanley W.	Navy	Philadelphia College of Pharmacy	KIA March 26, 1945; naval fighter pilot on aircraft carrier
Praedzik (Prawdzik)	Melvin A.		Connecticut	Killed in Italy
Prelutzky	George		St. Louis College of Pharmacy	
Price	Jack C.	AAF		Killed in an air crash in the Pacific in 1945
Procopio	Salvatore F.		Rutgers	KIA Battle of the Bulge
Rafferty	Michael A.	Army	West Virginia	Killed in action in Belgium
Redden	Paul W.	AAF	Oregon	Tail gunner—only member of the crew to be killed over Germany on July 7, 1944
Rerube	Edmund	Navy	Massachusetts College of Pharmacy	KIA on Iwo Jima
Rosin	Henry (Harry)	Army	Philadelphia College of Pharmacy	Died in service December 9, 1942
Rubin	Edward S.	Army	Philadelphia College of Pharmacy	Died in service August 15, 1943

Last Name	First Name, Middle Name	Service	School	Comment
Salyabongse	Somborgse	UN, OSS	Philadelphia College of Pharmacy	Operating behind enemy lines in Indo-China; executed when captured by the Japanese
Samwel	Daniel W. Jr.		Purdue	
Schoettel	John Fred	Marines	Washington	KIA in Guam— August 16, 1944
Shapiro	Paul	Army	Connecticut	Killed in the Mediterranean
Shatrwka	John Peter	AAF	Wisconsin	
Skelton	Donald R.	Army	Purdue	
Sotier	Charles Reis		St. Louis College of Pharmacy	
Spare	Frank B.	Navy	Philadelphia College of Pharmacy	October 1944 in the South Pacific
Sparks	Charles P.	AAF	Purdue	KIA over Germany, October 15, 1944
Steele	Wayne M.	AAF	Ohio State	KIA in action over England while on combat duty April 21, 1944
Stephenson	Edward Vassar	Marines	North Carolina	KIA at Iwo Jima while leading an attack on Motoyama Airfield #2, March 4, 1945
Stevenson	Harold M.	Army	Oregon	Captured at the fall of Bataan. On a Japanese prison ship sunk by a U.S. sub
Sullivan	Wayne H.	AAF	Cincinnati	KIA shot down over Cesena, northern Italy
Tashjian	Dickran		Fordham	Italy December 29, 1944

Last Name	First Name, Middle Name	Service	School	Comment
Thompson	John Ward	Army	Montana	KIA in the Philippines
Toupin	William A.	AAF	Ohio State	Africa December 24, 1942
Voyles	Charles	AAF	Butler	KIA over Weissenfels, Germany, on November 5, 1944
Wallace	John O.	Army	Medical College of Virginia	
Welde	Charles D.	AAF	Ohio State	Germany August 15, 1944
Wilkins	Raymond Harrell		North Carolina	KIA November 2, 1943
Wilson	Douglas		Massachusetts College of Pharmacy	Killed in training accident in 1941
Ziel	Glen Warren	Army		Killed in jeep wreck in Czechoslovakia

Notes

Preface

1. Worthen, D.B. and Smith, M.C. (1995). "When Pharmacy Went to War." *Pharmacy Times,* 61(7):35, 40, 42.
2. Mamet, Harvey S. Personal correspondence, September 11, 1995 and October 3, 1995.

Chapter 1

1. Evans, C.H. (1941). "Presidential Address." *Journal of the American Pharmaceutical Association,* Scientific Edition, 30:453-464.
2. Wilder, T. (1938). *Our Town.* New York: Harper and Brothers.
3. Nixon R.B. Jr. (1941). *Corner Druggist.* New York: Prentice-Hall, pp. vii-viii.
4. Shine, J. J. (1940). "The Prescription Volume in the Average Independent Drug Store." *Journal of the American Pharmaceutical Association,* Practical Pharmacy Edition, 1:127-129.
5. Eli Lilly and Company (1941). *A Lilly Digest of the 1941 Statements of 404 Retail Drug Stores,* Tenth Annual Edition. Indianapolis: Eli Lilly and Company.
6. Evans, C.H. (1941). "Presidential Installation Address." *Journal of the American Pharmaceutical Association,* Scientific Edition, 30:370-373.
7. Evans, "Presidential Address," p. 457.
8. American Association of Colleges of Pharmacy (1941). "Report of the Executive Committee." *American Journal of Pharmaceutical Education,* 526-527.
9. Anonymous (1938). "American Council on Pharmaceutical Education." *Journal of the American Pharmaceutical Association,* 27:64-65.
10. Anonymous (1939). "American Council on Pharmaceutical Education." *Journal of the American Pharmaceutical Association,* 28:806-809.
11. Flynn, G.Q. (1993). *The Draft, 1940-1973.* Lawrence: University Press of Kansas, pp. 1-53.
12. Perrett, G. (1985). *Days of Sadness, Years of Triumph: The American People, 1939-1945.* Madison: University of Wisconsin Press, p. 39.
13. Kendig, H.E. (1941). "The Pharmacist, the Pharmacy Student, and the Draft." *American Journal of Pharmaceutical Education,* 5:253-254.
14. Fisher, A.B. (1992). *A Half Century of Service to Pharmacy, 1942-1992.* Rockville, MD: American Foundation for Pharmaceutical Education, p. 3.
15. Buerki, R.A. (1977). "Pharmacy Extension Services at Purdue in the 1930's." *Pharmacy in History,* 19:79-88.

16. Dretzka, S.H. (1941). "Continuation Study for Pharmacists." *Journal of the American Pharmaceutical Association,* Scientific Edition, 30:529-531.

17. [Fischelis, R.P.] (1941). "The Shortage (?) of Pharmacists." *The New Jersey Journal of Pharmacy,* 14:6-7.

18. Kendig, H.E. (1942). "Committee on Status of Pharmacists in Government Service." *Journal of the American Pharmaceutical Association,* Scientific Edition, 31:393-399.

19. Evans, C.H. (1941). "President's Address." *Journal of the American Pharmaceutical Association,* Scientific Edition, 30:344-350.

20. Henderson, M.L. (2002). *American Women Pharmacists: Contributions to the Profession.* Binghamton, NY: Pharmaceutical Products Press, p. 69.

21. Anonymous (1942). "1940 Census Study Shows 81,924 Pharmacists in Practice." *Journal of the American Pharmaceutical Association,* Practical Pharmacy Edition, 3:254-255.

22. Christensen, B.V. (1941). "In-Coming Presidential Address." *Journal of the American Pharmaceutical Association,* Scientific Edition, 30:482-486.

23. Anonymous (1941). "Committee of Resolutions." *Journal of the American Pharmaceutical Association,* Scientific Edition, 30:547-548.

24. Anonymous (1941). "National Association Boards of Pharmacy." *Journal of the American Pharmaceutical Association,* Scientific Edition, 30:437-438.

25. Swain, R.L. (1941). "Committee on Modernization of Pharmacy Laws." *Journal of the American Pharmaceutical Association,* Scientific Edition, 30:489-490.

26. Fischelis, R P. (1941). "Food and Drug Legislation." *Journal of the American Pharmaceutical Association,* Scientific Edition, 30:528-529.

27. U.S. Civilian Production Administration (1969). *Industrial Mobilization for War: History of the War Production Board and Predecessor Agencies, 1940-1945.* Volume 1: *Program and Administration.* New York: Greenwood Press, p. 157 (a reprint of the GPO report of 1947).

28. Ehlke, E.E. "Lest We Forget." Memories Project Files.

Chapter 2

1. Kendig, H.E. (1942). Letter to Rudolph A. Kuever and Charles H. Rogers January 20. Archives of the American Pharmaceutical Association Foundation, Washington, DC.

2. American Council on Pharmaceutical Education (1942). List of Accredited Colleges of Pharmacy in the United States of America, April 1.

3. National Pharmaceutical Syllabus Committee (1932). *The Pharmaceutical Syllabus: Outlining the Course of Instruction for the Degree of Batchelor of Science in Pharmacy (B.S. Phar.),* Fourth Edition, p. 11.

4. Anonymous (1943). "Constitution and By-Laws of the American Association of Colleges of Pharmacy." *American Journal of Pharmaceutical Education,* 7:622-632.

5. Muldoon, H. (1944). "Who Will Teach Them?" *American Journal of Pharmaceutical Education,* 8:102-104.

6. Anonymous (1944). "Annual Report of the American Council of Pharmaceutical Education." *American Journal of Pharmaceutical Education,* 8:598-613.

7. DuMez, A.G. (1945). "Report on Need for Graduate Work in Pharmaceutical Subjects Prepared for the American Foundation for Pharmaceutical Education." *American Journal of Pharmaceutical Education,* 9:363-370.

8. Anonymous (1946). "Doctor Kidder Returns to Fordham." *The Fordham Pharmacist,* 4(February): 1-2.

9. Christensen, B.V. (n.d.). "Letter to Dean A. Ziefle." Ohio State University Archives, RG 20/1/4 "XYZ Miscellaneous Correspondence" 1941-1943.

10. Lewis, H.B. (1942). "Letter Summarizing College of Pharmacy Activities in the War Effort." October 22. Bentley Library Bimu C81 2 Box 2.

11. White, A.I. (1996). *The History of the Washington State University College of Pharmacy, 1891-1991.* Pullman, WA: College of Pharmacy, pp. 102-103.

12. Netz, C.V. (1971). *History of the University of Minnesota College of Pharmacy, 1892-1970.* Minneapolis: University of Minnesota College of Pharmacy, p. 93.

13. Knoll, H.B. (1947). "1941-1945: A Record of the University in War Years." *The Archives of Purdue,* (October):167-169.

14. Buerki, R.A. (1988). "Meeting the Continuing Education Challenge: The Association's Response, 1912-1965." *American Journal of Pharmaceutical Education,* 52:358-371.

15. Anonymous (1942). "Report of the Executive Committee." *American Journal of Pharmaceutical Education,* 6:504-506.

16. Anonymous (1942). "Survey Shows Serious Drop in Pharmacy Students at Most Western Institutions." *Pacific Drug Review,* (December):22-23.

17. Braucher, C.L. Memories Project Files.

18. Anonymous (1943). "Steps Taken to Increase Numbers of Pharmacy Students." *NARD Journal,* July 5:1064.

19. Anonymous (1944). "Special Meeting of the Executive Committee." *American Journal of Pharmaceutical Education,* 8:263.

20. Clark, H.E. Memories Project Files.

21. Kuever, R.A. (1942). "President's Bulletin Number 5." *American Journal of Pharmaceutical Education,* 6:137-138.

22. Kuever, R.A. (1942). "President's Bulletin Number 6." *American Journal of Pharmaceutical Education,* 6:139-142.

23. Barrett, L.B. (1942). "What Is to Be Gained by Speeding up the Educational Program?" *American Journal of Pharmaceutical Education,* 6:255-258.

24. Kuever, "President's Bulletin Number 6."

25. DuMez, A.G. (1942). "Letter to the Editor." *American Journal of Pharmaceutical Education,* 6:273-275.

26. Anonymous (1942). "Report of the Executive Committee." *American Journal of Pharmaceutical Education,* 6:509-512.

27. Anonymous (1942). "Policy of the American Council on Pharmaceutical Education with Regard to the Acceleration of the Course in Pharmacy for the Duration

of the War Emergency." *American Journal of Pharmaceutical Education,* 6:290-291.

28. *Proceedings of the 39th Annual Convention of the National Association of Boards of Pharmacy* (1942). August 17-18.

29. Kuever, R.A. (1943). "Our Experience with Intensified Courses of Study." *American Journal of Pharmaceutical Education,* 7:72-75.

30. Katsin, C.H. Memories Project Files.

31. U.S. Selective Service (1942). Selective Training and Service Act of 1940, as amended and regulations. Activity and Occupation Bulletin No. 33-6.

32. Anonymous (1943). "Gleanings from the Editor's Mail." *American Journal of Pharmaceutical Education,* 7:394.

33. The American Council on Pharmaceutical Education (1943). "Statement of Further Changes in Policy and Standards Made Necessary by the War Emergency." *American Journal of Pharmaceutical Education,* 7:409-411.

34. Bowers, R.A. and Cowen, D.L. (1991). *The Rutgers University College of Pharmacy: A Centennial History.* New Brunswick: Rutgers University Press, pp. 107-108.

35. Fischelis, R.P. (n.d.). "Letter to Charles H. Rogers." American Institute of History of Pharmacy Collection housed at the Wisconsin Historical Society, Madison, Wisconsin, Mss 619, Box 133, Folder 14.

36. Anonymous (1943). "Summary of Proceeding of the 1943 Meeting." *American Journal of Pharmaceutical Education,* 7:451.

37. Adams, A.L. (1943). "A Message from the President of the National Association of Boards of Pharmacy." *American Journal of Pharmaceutical Education,* 7:429-430.

38. Anonymous (1943). Proceedings of the 40th Annual Convention of the National Association of Boards of Pharmacy. September 9-10, pp. 138-139.

39. Dargavel, J.W. (1943). "Victory for Pharmacy." *American Journal of Pharmaceutical Education,* 7:560-561.

40. Anonymous (1944). "American Council on Pharmaceutical Education." *American Journal of Pharmaceutical Education,* 8:602.

41. Anonymous (1943). "Acceleration, Accreditation, and Licensure by Examination and Reciprocity." *American Journal of Pharmaceutical Education,* 7:588-589.

42. Lyman, R. (1943). "The Editor's Page." *American Journal of Pharmaceutical Education,* 7:564-569.

43. Little, E. (1944). "Some Further Thoughts on the Twenty-Four-Month Four-Term Program." *American Journal of Pharmaceutical Education,* 8:99-102.

44. Rogers, C.H. (1944). "Should Acceleration Be Continued?" *American Journal of Pharmaceutical Education,* 8:176-181.

45. Quintana, B.A. Memory Project Files.

46. Christensen, B.V. (1943). "Letter to J. G. Beard." March 31. Ohio State University Archives PG 20/a/1 "B Miscellaneous" 1939-1952.

47. Rogers, C.H. and Johnson, P.O. (1944). "Comparative Achievements of Accelerated and Non-Accelerated Groups of Students in the College of Pharmacy of

the University of Minnesota." *American Journal of Pharmaceutical Education,* 8:433-438.

48. Lee, C.O. (1945). "A Critical Evaluation of the Accelerated Program." *American Journal of Pharmaceutical Education,* 9:377-386.

49. Anonymous (1944). "American Council on Pharmaceutical Education." *American Journal of Pharmaceutical Education,* 8:602-603.

50. Lewis, H.B. (1942). "To the President of the University." Academic Year 1941-1942 Report. Bentley Historical Library Bimu C81 2 Box 2.

51. Philadelphia College of Pharmacy and Science (n.d.). "Women in Science During the War . . . and After" [recruitment brochure].

52. Henderson, M.L. (2002). *American Women Pharmacists: Contributions to the Profession.* Binghamton, NY: Pharmaceutical Products Press, pp. 69-70.

53. "The Woman Pharmacist" (1944). *New Jersey Journal of Pharmacy,* 17(May): cover 2 [advertisement].

54. "Your Daughter's Education" (1944). *New Jersey Journal of Pharmacy,* 17(April): cover 2 [advertisement].

55. Oregon State Pharmaceutical Association (1943). "For Women, Pharmacy Is an Ideal Vocation." Brochure.

56. Nekrassoff, L.H. Memories Project Files.

57. Anonymous (1944). "Women in Pharmacy [editorial]." *Pacific Drug Review,* (January):21.

58. Anonymous (1942). "College of Pharmacy, University of California." *Pacific Drug Review,* (May):72.

59. Anonymous (1942). "College of Pharmacy, University of Washington." *Pacific Drug Review,* (October):62.

60. Anonymous (1942). "College of Pharmacy, University of Southern California." *Pacific Drug Review,* (November):75.

61. O'Brien, R.W. (1949). *The College Nisei.* Palo Alto, CA: Pacific Books, pp. 135-139.

62. Daniels, R. (1993). *Prisoners Without Trial: Japanese Americans in World War II.* New York: Hill and Wang, pp. 129-130.

63. Anonymous (1942). "Nisei Students Win Many Awards at Washington U." *Pacific Citizen,* June 4.

64. University of California San Francisco (1985). *Pharmacy Alumni Association Newsletter,* spring, pp. 1-8.

65. O'Brien, *The College Nisei,* pp. 135-139.

66. Dickinson, V. Memories Project Files.

67. Anonymous (1944). "A Commemorative Album. "University of Nebraska-Lincoln Nisei Reunion," University of Nebraska, November 4-5.

68. Barrett, L. (1943). "Some Post-War Problems of Pharmaceutical Education." *American Journal of Pharmaceutical Education,* 7:155-160.

69. Anonymous (1943). "Report of the Committee on Long Range Program of Policy." *American Journal of Pharmaceutical Education,* 7:602-611.

70. Christensen, B.V. (1944). "Major Issues Confronting Post-War Pharmaceutical Education." *American Journal of Pharmaceutical Education,* 8:182-185.

71. Newton, H.C. (1944). "Editorials: Post-War Programs for Pharmaceutical Education." *American Journal of Pharmaceutical Education*, 8:231-232.

72. Wilson, R.C. (1945). "A Study of the Post-War Problems Confronting Pharmaceutical Education by the Committee on Post-War Planning." *American Journal of Pharmaceutical Education*, 9:59-130.

73. Wilson, R.C. (1944). "Report of the Committee on Post-War Planning." *American Journal of Pharmaceutical Education*, 8:623-629.

74. Fisher, A.B. (1992). *A Half Century of Service to Pharmacy, 1942-1992.* Rockville, MD: The American Foundation for Pharmaceutical Education, pp. 1-2.

75. Anonymous (1942). "Report of the American Foundation for Pharmaceutical Education, August 1942." *American Journal of Pharmaceutical Education*, 6:552-553.

76. Anonymous (1944). "Report of Representatives to American Foundation for Pharmaceutical Education." *American Journal of Pharmaceutical Education*, 8:447.

77. Rogers, E.S. (1944). "The Objectives of the American Foundation for Pharmaceutical Education." *American Journal of Pharmaceutical Education*, 8:316-327.

78. Anonymous (1944). "Report of the American Association of Colleges of Pharmacy Representatives to the American Foundation for Pharmaceutical Education." *American Journal of Pharmaceutical Education*, 8:572-575.

79. Anonymous (1945). "Editorial." *American Journal of Pharmaceutical Education*, 9:261.

80. Lyman, R. (1944). "The Editor's Page." *American Journal of Pharmaceutical Education*, 8:242-245.

81. Fisher, *A Half Century of Service to Pharmacy*, pp. 89-95.

82. Anonymous (1944). "American Foundation for Pharmaceutical Education." *American Journal of Pharmaceutical Education*, 8:402-403.

83. Anonymous (1942). "Report of the Committee on the Status of Pharmacists in the Government Service." *American Journal of Pharmaceutical Education*, 6:574-580.

84. Anonymous (1942). "Federal Aid for Pharmacy Students in Accelerated Courses." *American Pharmaceutical Association Bulletin* (1941-1942) No. 42, July 15.

85. Anonymous (1944). "Loans Given 438 Pharmacy Students by Government." *Journal of the American Pharmaceutical Association*, Practical Pharmacy Edition, 5:16.

86. Anonymous (1945). "Kickoff Meeting to Precede Drive for Funds for College." *O.V.D.A. Review*, 5(7):10.

87. Christensen, B.V. (1944). "Major Issues Confronting Post-War Pharmaceutical Education." *American Journal of Pharmaceutical Education*, 8:182-185.

88. Lyman, R. (1944). "The Editor's Page." *American Journal of Pharmaceutical Education*, 8:372.

89. Rowe, T.D. (1945). "Refresher Courses in Dispensing Pharmacy for Returning Registered Pharmacists." *American Journal of Pharmaceutical Education*, 9:22-26.

90. Magee, J.C. quoted in anonymous (1942). "Report of the Executive Committee." *American Journal of Pharmaceutical Education*, 6:510-511.

91. Anonymous (1943). "Report of the Committee on Educational and Membership Standards." *American Journal of Pharmaceutical Education,* 7:497-501.

92. Anonymous (1944). "Report of the Committee on College Credit for Military Experience." *American Journal of Pharmaceutical Education,* 8:277-281.

93. Anonymous (1944). "Report of the Special Joint Committee to Study Nature and Extent of Pharmacy Training in the Armed Forces." *American Journal of Pharmaceutical Education,* 8:586-594.

94. Anonymous (1944). "Annual Report of the American Council on Pharmaceutical Education, Inc." *American Journal of Pharmaceutical Education,* 8:604-606.

95. Fischelis, R.P. (1945). *American Journal of Pharmaceutical Education,* 9:405.

Chapter 3

1. Selective Training and Service Act of 1940, U.S. Statutes at Large. 76th Congress, Third Session, 1939-1941. Volume 54, part 1. *Public Laws and Reorganization Plans,* pp. 885-897.

2. Flynn, G.Q. (1993). *The Draft, 1940-1973.* Lawrence: University Press of Kansas, pp. 1-53.

3. Ketchum, R.M. (1989). *The Borrowed Years 1938-1942: America on the Way to War.* New York: Random House, p. 646.

4. Elliott, E.C. (1950). *General Report of the Pharmaceutical Survey 1946-1949.* Washington, DC: American Council on Education, pp. 31-32.

5. Kendig, H.E. (1941). "The Pharmacist, the Pharmacy Student, and the Draft." *American Journal of Pharmaceutical Education,* 5:253-255.

6. Brown, F.J. (1941). "The Problems of Selective Service As They Affect Students of Pharmacy." *American Journal of Pharmaceutical Education,* 5:473-483.

7. Anonymous (1941). "Editorial." *New Jersey Journal of Pharmacy,* 14(March):6-7.

8. Kuever, R.A. (1941). "Pharmacy and Our National Defense." *Northwestern Druggist,* July:15, 32.

9. Anonymous (1942). "Editorial." *Virginia Pharmacist,* 26:4.

10. Anonymous (1942). "81,924 Pharmacists in Practice: 1940 Census Study Shows." *Journal of the American Pharmaceutical Association,* Practical Pharmacy Edition, 3:254-255.

11. American Pharmaceutical Association (1942). "Summary of Pharmaceutical Personnel Statistics for 1940." *American Pharmaceutical Association Bulletin.* No. 38-1941-1942, June 23.

12. Hershey, L.B. (1942). "Memorandum to All State Directors (I-405) and Local Board Release (115)." Selective Service System, March 16.

13. Dean, N.D. (1943). "Letter to Minnesota State Pharmaceutical Association, January 13, 1943." American Institute of History of Pharmacy Collection housed at the Wisconsin Historical Society, Madison, Wisconsin, Manuscript 619, Box 71, folder 4.

14. Fischelis, R.P. and Fiero, G. (1943). "Civilian Requirements for Pharmacists." *NARD Journal,* 65(October 4):1570, 1572, 1574.

15. Anonymous (1944). "Selective Service Officer Thinks There Are Too Many Pharmacies." *NARD Journal,* 66(May 1):1252.

16. Lemon, A.B. (1944). "Too Many Pharmacies?" *New York State Pharmacist,* (March):10.

17. Yocum, J.C. and Arnold, S. (1943). *Pharmacy Manpower.* Columbus, OH: Ohio Bureau of Business Research, The Ohio State University.

18. Hershey, L.B. (1941). "Memorandum to All State Directors (I-10): Classification of Registrants in Training or Preparation." Selective Service System, March 7.

19. Hershey, L.B. (1941). "Memorandum to All State Directors (I-62): Occupational Deferment of Students and Other Necessary Men in Certain Specialized Professional Fields (III)." Selective Service System, April 22.

20. Hershey, L.B. (1942). "Memorandum to All State Directors (I-405) and Local Board Release (115)." Selective Service System, March 16.

21. Christensen, B.V. (1942). "Letter to H.C. Newton." November 10. Ohio State Archives, Record Group 20/a/3 "N. Miscellaneous Correspondence" 1939-1951.

22. Committee on War Activities of the American Pharmaceutical Association (1942). "Letter to Edward C. Elliott." December 1. American Institute of History of Pharmacy Collection housed at the Wisconsin Historical Society, Madison, Wisconsin, Mss 619, Box 71, Folder 4.

23. War Activities Committee, American Pharmaceutical Association (1943). "Meeting Summary." February 13. 2 pp. American Institute of History of Pharmacy Collection housed at the Wisconsin Historical Society, Madison, Wisconsin, Mss 619, Box 71, Folder 4.

24. War Activities Committee (1943). "Letter to Henry L. Stimson." March 1. American Institute of History of Pharmacy Collection housed at the Wisconsin Historical Society, Madison, Wisconsin, Mss 619, Box 71, Folder 4.

25. DuMez, A.G. (1943). "Report of the War Emergency Advisory Committee." *American Journal of Pharmaceutical Education,* 7:515-523.

26. Anonymous (1943). "A Brief in Support of the Continued Classification of Pharmacy As an Essential Activity Under Health and Welfare Service, the Continued Deferment of Pharmacists, and a Provision for the Training of an Adequate Number of Pharmacists." May 1. American Institute of History of Pharmacy Collection housed at the Wisconsin Historical Society, Madison, Wisconsin, Mss 619, Box 71, Folder 4.

27. Anonymous (1943). "Selective Service Announces New Student Deferment Policy." *Journal of the American Pharmaceutical Association,* Practical Pharmacy Edition, 4:51-52.

28. Anonymous (1943). "Deferment of Students." *Virginia Pharmacist,* 27:89.

29. War Emergency Advisory Committee (1943). "Report." *Journal of the American Pharmaceutical Association,* Scientific Edition, 32:435-436.

30. Fischelis, R.P. (1943). "Letter to Rufus Lyman." July 3. American Institute of History of Pharmacy Collection housed at the Wisconsin Historical Society, Madison, Wisconsin, Mss 619, Box 71, Folder 4.

31. Christensen, B.V. (1944). "Letter to Robert Swain." January 27. Ohio State University Archives, RG20/a/1 "Drug Topics 1941-1945."

32. Flynn, G.Q. (1993). *The Draft,* p. 79.

33. Selective Training and Service Act of 1940 (Sec 5. (e)) U.S. Statutes at Large, 76th Congress, Third Session, Volume 54, part 1. Public Laws and Reorganization Plans, p. 888.

34. Executive Order, Selective Service Regulations, Volume III, Classification and Selection (#8560), Paragraph 351.

35. Selective Service Commission (1943). "Activity and Occupation Bulletin No. 32." Issued March 1 and amended May 29.

36. Anonymous (1942). "Oregon Advises Draft Boards." *NARD Journal,* 64(July 5):1076.

37. Powers, D.B. Memory Project Files.

38. Selective Service Commission (1943). "Selective Service Bulletin 56-43." Issued June 16 as cited in the second meeting, Robert P. Fischelis Papers, American Institute of History of Pharmacy Collection housed at the Wisconsin Historical Society, Madison, Wisconsin, Mss 619, Box 118, Folder 2, p. 4.

39. Anonymous (1942). "New Hampshire Editorial Page." *Apothecary,* (March):22.

40. Anonymous (1943). "Associations Name Selective Service Advisors." *NARD Journal,* 65(July 5): 1078.

41. APhA Advisory Committees (1943). Selective Service. Archives of the American Pharmaceutical Association Foundation, Washington, DC.

42. Lemon, A.B. (1943). "Report of the Advisory Committee to Selective Service." New York State Pharmaceutical Association 65th Annual Convention June 16-17. Archives of the American Pharmaceutical Association Foundation, Washington, DC.

43. Shine, J.J. (1943). "Letter to Jennings Murphy." July 30. Archives of the American Pharmaceutical Association Foundation, Washington, DC.

44. Kleber, V. (1948). *Selective Service In Illinois 1940-1947.* Springfield: State of Illinois, p. 143.

45. First Meeting of the Pharmacy Advisory Committee to Selective Service, Robert P. Fischelis Papers, American Institute of History of Pharmacy Collection housed at the Wisconsin Historical Society, Madison, Wisconsin, Mss 619, Box 118, Folder 2, p. 1.

46. Second Meeting of the Pharmacy Advisory Committee to Selective Service, Robert P. Fischelis Papers, American Institute of History of Pharmacy Collection housed at the Wisconsin Historical Society, Madison, Wisconsin, Madison, Mss 619, Box 118, Folder 2, p. 9.

47. Sixth Meeting of the Pharmacy Advisory Committee to Selective Service, Robert P. Fischelis Papers, American Institute of History of Pharmacy Collection housed at the Wisconsin Historical Society, Madison, Wisconsin, Mss 619, Box 118, Folder 2, p. 24.

48. Twelfth Meeting of the Pharmacy Advisory Committee to Selective Service, Robert P. Fischelis Papers, American Institute of History of Pharmacy Collection housed at the Wisconsin Historical Society, Madison, Wisconsin, Mss 619, Box 118, Folder 2, pp. 49-50.

49. Second Meeting of the Pharmacy Advisory Committee to Selective Service, Robert P. Fischelis Papers, American Institute of History of Pharmacy Collection housed at the Wisconsin Historical Society, Madison, Wisconsin, Mss 619, Box 118, Folder 2, p. 10.

50. Ninth Meeting of the Pharmacy Advisory Committee to Selective Service, Robert P. Fischelis Papers, American Institute of History of Pharmacy Collection housed at the Wisconsin Historical Society, Madison, Wisconsin, Mss 619, Box 118, Folder 2, p. 40.

51. Tenth Meeting of the Pharmacy Advisory Committee to Selective Service, Robert P. Fischelis Papers, American Institute of History of Pharmacy Collection housed at the Wisconsin Historical Society, Madison, Wisconsin, Mss 619, Box 118, Folder 2, p. 45.

52. Seventh Meeting of the Pharmacy Advisory Committee to Selective Service, Robert P. Fischelis Papers, American Institute of History of Pharmacy Collection housed at the Wisconsin Historical Society, Madison, Wisconsin, Mss 619, Box 118, Folder 2, p. 29.

53. Eighth Meeting of the Pharmacy Advisory Committee to Selective Service, Robert P. Fischelis Papers, American Institute of History of Pharmacy Collection housed at the Wisconsin Historical Society, Madison, Wisconsin, Mss 619, Box 118, Folder 2, pp. 36-37.

54. Eighth Meeting of the Pharmacy Advisory Committee to Selective Service, Robert P. Fischelis Papers, American Institute of History of Pharmacy Collection housed at the Wisconsin Historical Society, Madison, Wisconsin, Mss 619, Box 118, Folder 2, p. 34.

55. Curran, F.F. (Ed.) (1995). *Keeping in Touch: Letters from Alumni and Students to the Philadelphia College of Pharmacy and Science During World War II.* Philadelphia: Philadelphia College of Pharmacy and Science, p. 63.

56. Eighth Meeting of the Pharmacy Advisory Committee to Selective Service, Robert P. Fischelis Papers, American Institute of History of Pharmacy Collection housed at the Wisconsin Historical Society, Madison, Wisconsin, Mss 619, Box 118, Folder 2, p. 34.

57. Ninth Meeting of the Pharmacy Advisory Committee to Selective Service, Robert P. Fischelis Papers, American Institute of History of Pharmacy Collection housed at the Wisconsin Historical Society, Madison, Wisconsin, Mss 619, Box 118, Folder 2, p. 41.

58. Anonymous (1945). *New Jersey Journal of Pharmacy,* 15(May):8-9.

59. Ohio State University (1943). "University Credit for Military Service." March 12. OSU Archives RG20/a/1 "Faculty Council 1938-1947."

60. Ford, M.M. Correspondence 1940-1947.Ohio State University Archives RG 20/a/1/.

61. Anonymous (1942). "Special Examination Is Held for Those Entering the Service." *North Western Druggist,* (August):55.

62. Segel, M. Memories Project Files.

63. NABP (1942). Proceedings of the 39th Annual Convention of the National Association of Boards of Pharmacy, August 17-18, pp. 67-76.

64. NABP (1943). Proceedings of the 40th Annual Convention of the National Association of Boards of Pharmacy, September 9-10, pp. 95-108.

65. Anonymous (1943). "Requirements for Reciprocal Registration." *American Journal of Pharmaceutical Education,* 7:244-246.

66. Pickard, J.F. Memories Project Files.

67. Michigan State Board Minutes (1944). January 12. Michigan State Archives RG82-42 Box 1, folder 2.

68. Michigan State Board Minutes (9145).October 30. Michigan State Archives RG82-42 Box 1, folder 3.

Chapter 4

1. Evans, C.H. (1941). "President's Address." *Journal of the American Pharmaceutical Association,* Scientific Edition, 30:455-457.

2. Anonymous (194). "War and the Druggist: A Report from Druggists on the Atlantic and Pacific 'Borders.'" *NARD Journal,* 64(January 1):15-16, 57.

3. Anonymous (1942). *Drug Topics,* (April 6):4, 12.

4. Baehr, G. (1942). "Civilian Defense and the Role of the Drugstore." *American Druggist,* 105(February):32-33, 96.

5. Hutchins, H. (1942). "Drugstores Ruled Out by the Office of Civilian Defense and Here's Why." *American Druggist,* 105(February):30-31, 96.

6. Anonymous (1942). "Manual for Pharmacists in Civilian Defense." *Journal of the American Pharmaceutical Association,* Practical Pharmacy Edition, 3:4-12.

7. Anonymous (1942). "An Open Letter to Cincinnati Druggists." *The O.V.D.A Review,* (February):1, 6-7.

8. Anonymous (1942). "Druggists Across the Nation Prepare to Go All-Out for Civilian Defense." *NARD Journal,* 64(March 19):378-380, 410, 414.

9. *Industrial Mobilization for War: History of the War Production Board and Predecessor Agencies 1940-1945* (1947). Volume 1: *Program and Administration.* Washington DC: GPO. Reprinted by Greenwood Press, New York, 1969, p. 426.

10. Overy, R. (1996). *Why the Allies Won.* New York: W. W. Norton, pp. 180-207.

11. Cook, R.B. (1942). "War Activities of Pharmacists." *Journal of the American Pharmaceutical Association,* Practical Pharmacy Edition, 3:334-338.

12. Cohen, S. (1991). *V For Victory: America's Home Front During World War II.* Missoula, MT: Pictorial Histories Publishing Company, pp. 60-61.

13. Rennick, D. (1942). "$22,725,720 in War Savings Stamps Have Been Sold in U.S. Drugstores." *Drug Topics,* 20(April 6):4, 12.

14. Anonymous (1942). "Editorial." *The Apothecary,* 53(April):8.

15. Anonymous (1942). "Defense Stamp Sales Drive by Drug Industry." *Southeastern Drug Journal,* 45(May):9.

16. Anonymous (1942). "Druggists Get Behind Bullet Drive." *NARD Journal,* 64(May 7):586-589.

17. Anonymous (1942). "Behind the Men Behind the Guns" [editorial]. Hearst Newspapers (including *New York Journal-American*) May 4, 1942; reprinted in *American Druggist,* 105(June):25.

18. Anonymous (1942). "May War Stamp and Bond Drive by Druggists Exceed $7,253,362.35." *American Druggist,* 106(July):32-35.

19. Rennick, D. (1942). "$22,725,720 in War Savings Stamps."

20. Anoymous (1943). "Druggist Successful in Build-A-Sub Campaign." *NARD Journal,* 65(September 20):1432.

21. Anonymous (1944). "Queens Pharmacists Launch Submarine." *New York State Pharmacist,* (March):16.

22. Anonymous (1944). "Queens County Druggist Sponsored Submarine." *NARD Journal,* 66(March 20):489.

23. Anonymous (1943). "Flying Ambulances and Other Campaigns." *The Apothecary,* 55(November):4.

24. Anonymous (1944). "NARD Accepts Ambulance Plane Drive." *The Apothecary,* 56(January):7.

25. Anonymous (1944). "Drug organizations Urged to Sponsor Ambulance Planes Through Sales of War Bonds." *NARD Journal,* 66(January 3):24, 57, 60.

26. Anonymous (1944). "Druggists Buy Eight Planes." *The Arkansas Druggist,* 6(March):3.

27. Anonymous (1944). "Druggists Sell Enough War Bonds to Build 54 Ambulance Planes." *NARD Journal,* 66(July 3):1152-1153.

28. Anonymous (1944). "Druggists in 5th War Loan." *The Arkansas Druggist,* 6(May):12.

29. Anonymous (1944). "New York City Pharmacists Conduct Hospital Train Drive." *New York State Pharmacist,* (December):14.

30. Rodda, J.W. Memories Project Files.

31. Anonymous (1945). "Washington Druggists Will Sponsor LST Commanded by Local Pharmacist." *Pacific Drug Review,* 57(February):50.

32. Anonymous (1943). "'Back the Attack;' The Third War Loan Starts September 9." *American Druggist,* 108(September):56.

33. Anonymous (1945). "Druggists Cooperate in the Mighty 7th War Loan Drive." *American Druggist,* 111(June):55, 96.

34. U.S. Civilian Production Administration (1947). *Industrial Mobilization for War: History of the War Production Board and Predecessor Agencies 1940-1945.* Volume 1: *Program and Administration.* Washington, DC: GPO. Reprinted by Greenwood Press, New York, 1969, p. 157.

35. Anonymous (n.d.). "Why Save Tin Cans?" (Pub. no. 16-35774-1.) Washington, DC: GPO.

36. Anonymous (1942). "Druggists to Collect Collapsible Tin Tubes." *The Apothecary,* 54(February):9.

37. American Pharmaceutical Association (1942). "WPB Issues Tin Tube Order." *Bulletin* No. 20 (1941-1942). April 2.

38. Anonymous (1942). "Pharmacy's Tin Salvage Record." *Northwestern Druggist,* (December):21, 53.

39. Anonymous (1945). "Syrettes from Can Salvage." *Squibb Sales Bulletin,* (April 19):187.

40. Anonymous (1944). "Tin Tubes." *Carolina Journal of Pharmacy,* 25:37.

41. Ingram Shaving Cream (1945). Advertisement. *Northwestern Druggist,* 20(April):7.

42. Squibb Tooth Powder (1943). Advertisement. *The Apothecary,* 55(February):17.

43. Anonymous (1943). "Tin for Victory." *Northwestern Druggist,* (January):12.

44. Anonymous (1940). "Attempts to Dominate Quinine Industry." *Journal of the American Pharmaceutical Association,* Practical Pharmacy Edition, 1:454.

45. Anonymous (1942). "Monopoly over Malaria." *Medical Care,* 2:111-117.

46. War Production Board (1942). "War Production Board Quinine Order." *Bulletin of the National Formulary Committee,* 10(4):95-99.

47. War Production Board (1942). "Quinine Order Amended." *Bulletin of the National Formulary Committee,* 10(5):106-118.

48. War Production Board (1942). "WPB Revokes 50 Ounce Quinine Exemption." *Bulletin of the National Formulary Committee,* 10(7):163-167.

49. Anonymous (1942). "A Survey of Stocks of Cinchona Alkaloids on Hand in Original Containers in 1800 Retail Drugstores in the State of New Jersey as of July 1, 1942." Fischelis Files. American Institute of History of Pharmacy Collection housed at the Wisconsin Historical Society, Madison, Wisconsin, RG619 Box 135 File 5.

50. Kramer, J.E. (1943). "The Story of the Quinine Pool." *American Druggist,* 107(January):46, 86.

51. Defense Supplies Corporation Contract 56-P-83, Jan 15, 1943. Fischelis Files. American Institute of History of Pharmacy Collection housed at the Wisconsin Historical Society, Madison, Wisconsin RG 619 Box 91 File 5.

52. Anonymous (1942). "Send Your Quinine Off to War." *Journal of the American Pharmaceutical Association,* Practical Pharmacy Edition, 3:403-413.

53. Hajla, W.J. (1943). "The National Quinine Pool." *The Hospital Corps Quarterly,* 16(4):1-47.

54. Anonymous (1942). "60 Colleges Volunteer for Quinine Collection." *Drug Topics,* 20(December 7):3.

55. Anonymous (1943). "Collection of Quinine by State Highway Patrol Outstanding Success." *Carolina Journal of Pharmacy,* 24:262-263.

56. Christensen, B.V. (n.d.), Letter to Bevis, H. Ohio State University Archives, University Offices, "Bevis Letters 1940-1952" RG20/9/4.

57. Anonymous (1943). "Pharmacists Answering Call for Quinine." *Journal of the American Pharmaceutical Association,* Practical Pharmacy Edition, 4:5-14.

58. Anonymous (1943). "Snell Urges Oregonians to Give Quinine to Soldiers." *Pacific Drug Review,* 20(August):25.

59. Anonymous (1943). "Quinine Story Told on Air." *Journal of the American Pharmaceutical Association,* Practical Pharmacy Edition, 4:12-14.

60. Anonymous (1943). "National Pool Receives Presidential Quinine Gift." *Journal of the American Pharmaceutical Association,* Practical Pharmacy Edition, 4:170-171.

61. Anonymous (1943). "Quinine Pool Finishes War Job." *Journal of the American Pharmaceutical Association,* Practical Pharmacy Edition, 4:369-370.

62. Hajla, W.J. (1943). "The National Quinine Pool." *The Hospital Corps Quarterly,* 16(4):1-47.

63. Worthen, D.B. (1996). "The National Quinine Pool: When Quinine Went to War." *Pharmacy in History,* 38:143-147.

64. Moulton, G.A. (1944). "National Pharmacy Week Message." *Journal of the American Pharmaceutical Association,* Practical Pharmacy Edition, 5:260-261.

65. Flannery, M.A. (1996). "Smith Pharmacy in Burkesville, Kentucky: A Case Study in the Development of a Community Pharmacy." *The Register of the Kentucky Historical Society,* 94(4):396-402.

66. Glover, D.D. Memories Project Files.

Chapter 5

1. Jackson, R.A. and Worthen, D.B. (2002). "Retail Pharmacy Operations in World War II: A Profit and Loss Statement." *Pharmacy in History,* 44:131-141.

2. Anonymous (1942). *Southeastern Drug Journal,* 17(September):13-57.

3. Anonymous (1942). *American Professional Pharmacist,* 8:559-64, 594.

4. Joseph A. Hailer United Drug Company (1941). "Limitation on Shipments of 'Scarce' Drugs." Bulletin #412. Boston, Massachusetts, January 21.

5. Anonymous (1941). "Exports of Belladonna and Atropine Prohibited." *New Jersey Journal of Pharmacy,* 14(March):28.

6. Anonymous (1941). "Shortage of Materials." *New Jersey Journal of Pharmacy,* 14(October):8.

7. Newcomb, E.L. (1941). Letter to E. Fullerton Cook. October 21. Ohio State University Archives RG 20/1/l "Ergot 1941."

8. Anonymous (1941/1942). *NF Letter,* (4):13-14.

9. Anderson, L. and Higby, G.J. (1995). *The Spirit of Voluntarism: A Legacy of Commitment and Contribution, The United States Pharmacopoeia 1820-1995.* Rockville, MD: United States Pharmacopoeia, p. 520.

10. Anonymous (1942). "War Shortage of Drugs and Medical Appliances: Report of a Subcommittee of the Committee on Public Health Relations of the New York Academy of Medicine." *New York State Journal of Medicine,* 42:857, 916, 918, 920.

11. Powers, J.L. (1942). "War Problems of the National Formulary." *Proceedings of the American Drug Manufacturers Association 31st Annual Meeting,* May 4-7, pp. 139-143.

12. Merrill, E.C. (1942). "Immediate Problems and Trends Arising from War Effort in Pharmaceutical Manufacturing." *Bulletin of the National Formulary Committee,* 10(July):156-163.

13. Ibid.

14. Beeler, E.C., Steinmetz, C.A., and Green, M.W. (1943). "Report from the APhA Laboratory: Glycerin Replacement." *Bulletin of the National Formulary Committee,* 11(January-February):11-12.

15. Anonymous (1943). "Florida Drug World." *Southeastern Drug Journal,* 18(April):32.

16. Anonymous (1942). "Sugar Shortage Emphasizes Need for Druggists to Tighten Business Belts." *NARD Journal,* 64(February 5):190-191.

17. Pittenger, P.S. (1943). "The Essentiality of Sucrose for Medicinal Products." *Bulletin of the National Formulary Committee,* 11(July-August):133-143.

18. Anonymous (1943). "Castoria Stocks Recalled." *Southeastern Drug Journal,* 17(June):39.

19. Anonymous (1943). "Castoria Mystery Solved: Manufacture Is Resumed." *Southeastern Drug Journal,* 17(July):45.

20. Merrill, "Immediate Problems and Trends."

21. Olson, J. Memories Project Files.

22. Anonymous (1943). "Retail Pharmacy Profits in a War Year." *American Professional Pharmacist,* 9:572.

23. Anonymous (1943). "Mistura . . ." *Pacific Drug Review,* (July):16.

24. Anonymous (1943). "This Drug Business." *American Druggist,* 107(February):132.

25. Anonymous (1942). "National Officers Installed by Druggists; Sideline Merchandise Is Becoming Scarce." *Cincinnati Enquirer,* (August 25):10.

26. Miller, N.A. (1944). *Wartime Guide for Retail Druggists.* Economic Series 33. Chicago: Department of Commerce. Printed and Distributed by the National Association of Retail Druggists, pp. 30-33.

27. Biemersderfer, J. Memories Project Files.

28. Anonymous (1942). *Pacific Drug Review,* 54(May):42.

29. War Relocation Authority (1943). *Relocation of Japanese-Americans.* Washington, DC: War Relocation Authority.

30. Kitabayshi, S. (1997). Memories Project Correspondence.

31. Oral History Tamako (Inouye) Tokuda, with Louis Fiset December 9, 1998.

32. United States Department of War (1943). *Final Report: Japanese Evacuation from the West Coast 1942.* Washington, DC: GPO.

33. Michigan Board of Pharmacy (1944). Minutes, June 19. Michigan Archives RG 82-42 B1 f2.

34. Matsuda, B.S. Memories Project Files.

35. Miller, *Wartime Guide,* p. 35.

36. Shine, J.J. (1940). "The Prescription Volume in the Average Independent Drugstore." *Journal of the American Pharmaceutical Association,* Practical Pharmacy Edition, 1:127-129.

37. Eli Lilly and Company (1940). *Lilly Digest,* Ninth Annual Edition. Indianapolis: Eli Lilly and Company, p. 4.

38. Shine, J.J. (1940). "Prescription Volume."

39. Anonymous (1942). *Drug Topics,* 86(April 6):4, 12.

40. Anonymous (1942). American Professional Pharmacist, 8:560.

41. Rogers, Charles H. (1943). Letter to Edward G. Elliott [War Manpower Commission]. April 10. Kremers Files, American Institute of the History of Pharmacy, Madison, Wisconsin, Group 716 Box 4, folder 5.

42. Anonymous (1943). "Massachusetts Editorial." *The Apothecary,* (April):11.

43. Anonymous (1944). "Iowa News." *Northwestern Druggist,* (March):58.

44. Ebets, H. Memories Project Files.

45. Anonymous (1942). "War Damage Insurance." *New York State Pharmacist,* August:26.

46. Johnson, V.B. Memories Project Files.

47. Anonymous (1943). "Retail Pharmacy Profits in a War Year." *American Professional Pharmacist,* 9(September):570.

48. U.S. Department of Commerce (1946). *Statistical Abstract of the United States 1946.* Washington, DC: GPO, p. 952, Table 1043.

49. Anonymous (1942). "Drug-Store Profits in Wartime." *Southeastern Drug Journal,* 17(September):13.

50. Blum, J.M. (1976). *V Was for Victory.* New York: Harcourt Brace Jovanovich, p. 91.

51. Dr. West Toothbrushes (1943). Advertisements. *Saturday Evening Post,* (January 9):61 and (February 20):58.

52. Sal Hepatica (1943). Advertisement. *Saturday Evening Post,* (January 30):69.

53. Felter, W.C. (1943). "Bureau of Census Reports Show Big Drugstore Gain in Sales for 1943." *Pacific Drug Review,* (September):35-36.

54. Anonymous (1944). "Causes of Drugstore Closures Reviewed in NWDA Survey." *Pacific Drug Review,* 20(May):27, 40.

55. Anonymous (1943). "Mistura . . ." *Pacific Drug Review,* (January):16.

56. Anonymous (1943). "Shipping Space Saved by Compressing Napkins." *NARD Journal,* 65(July 5):1078.

57. Anonymous (1942). "Drugstore Profits in Wartime." *Southeastern Drug Journal,* 17(September):14.

58. Anonymous (1943). "Who Will Compound Them?" *The Apothecary,* (June):4.

59. Anonymous (1943). "Fewer Doctors—More Prescriptions." *The Merck Report,* (July):3.

60. Miller, *Wartime Guide,* p. 12.

61. Office of Price Administration (1942). "Maximum Price Regulation." Bulletin No.1. *Northwestern Druggist,* 20(June):58, 60, 62, 64, 66.

62. Anonymous (1943). *Pacific Drug Review,* (March):38.

63. Anonymous (1943). "Retail Pharmacy Profits in a War Year." *American Professional Pharmacist,* 9:573.

64. Jackson, R.A. and Worthen, D.B., "Retail Pharmacy Operations in World War II."

65. Fischelis, R.P. and Fiero, G. (1943). "The Civilian Requirements for Pharmacists." *NARD Journal,* 65(October 4):1570, 1572, 1574.

66. Anonymous (1943). "Excerpts from the Mail." *The New Jersey Journal of Pharmacy,* 16(December):24.

67. Elliott, E.C. (1950). *General Report of the Pharmaceutical Survey 1946-49.* Washington, DC: American Council on Education, pp. 135-137.

68. Anonymous (1943). "Tennessee Topics." *Southeastern Drug Journal,* 18(January):40.

69. Anonymous (1943). "Tennessee Topics." *Southeast Drug Journal,* 18(March):70.

70. Yocum, J.C. and Arnold, S. (1943). *Pharmacy Manpower.* Columbus: Ohio Bureau of Business Research, The Ohio State University.

71. Anonymous (1943). "Fifteen Percent of NY Pharmacists in Service." *NARD Journal,* 65 (August 2):1203.

72. Anonymous (1944). "Utah . . ." *Pacific Drug Review,* 56(December):73.

73. Anonymous (1943). "North Carolina: Strictly Personal." *Southeastern Drug Journal,* 18 (October):37.

74. Miller, *Wartime Guide* p. 35.

75. Hartlaub, G.S. Memories Project Files.

76. Rae, J.B. (1984). *The American Automobile Industry.* Boston: G.K. Hall & Company, p. xii.

77. Anonymous (1942). "Registered Pharmacists Wanted." *Carolina Journal of Pharmacy,* 23(December):381.

78. Anonymous (1943). "Some Tennessee Counties Have No Pharmacists." *NARD Journal,* 65(April 19):622.

79. Anonymous (1942). "Why Not Girl Pharmacists?" *Apothecary,* (April):47.

80. Anonymous (1943). "South Carolina Items." Southeast Drug Journal, 20(April):25.

81. "Help Wanted Ad" (1944). *ASHP Bulletin* 10(August):3.

82. Vescio, F. and Knabe, M. (1943). "Women and Wartime Pharmacy." *The Merck Report,* (July):8-9.

83. Anonymous (1943). "How Druggists Are Meeting the Manpower Shortage." *NARD Journal,* 65(May 17):733-734, 779.

84. Dolezal, V. Memories Project Files.

85. Curran, F.F. (1988). *Compounding WAS More Fun!!!* Frances F. Curran and Lambda Kappa Sigma, pp. 69-70.

86. Dretzka, S. (1934). "Will Men Be Supplanted by Women in Pharmacy?" *Northwestern Druggist,* (January):22, 57, 60.

87. Anonymous (1944). "1942 Survey of 13,382 Prescriptions." *American Druggist,* 110(November):68-69.

88. Ruedig, D.F. (1942). "The Prescription Business in Wartime." *North Western Druggist,* 20(August):21, 47, 53, 57, 59.

89. Burlage, H.M. (1944). "North Carolina Prescription Survey." *American Druggist,* 110(October):62-63.

90. Crossen, G.E. (1944). "How Much Compounding Skill Is Needed to Fill Today's Prescriptions?" *American Druggist,* 110(September):60-61.

91. Anonymous (1943). "A Brief in Support of the Continued Classification of Pharmacy As an Essential Activity Under Health and Welfare Service, the Continued Deferment of Pharmacists, and a Provision for the Training of an Adequate Number of Pharmacists." May 1. American Institute of History of Pharmacy Collection housed at the Wisconsin Historical Society, Madison, Wisconsin, Mss 619, Box 71, Folder 4.

92. Daniels, T.C. (1943). "American Born Japanese Graduates of College of Pharmacy Are Available." *Hospitals,* 17(May):93.

93. Proceedings of the Annual Convention of the National Association of Boards of Pharmacy (1945). Tables 7 and 8.

94. United States Department of Commerce (1950). *Statistical Abstract of the United States 1950,* p. 83.

96. American Hospital Association (1948). *American Hospital Directory Association* [survey data as of 1947], pp. C-5, C-32.

96. Templeton, L. (1942). "Hospital Pharmaceuticals During the War." *Hospitals,* 16(October):35-37.

97. Fischelis, R.P. and Mordell, J.S. (1943). "Effect of War Production Board Orders on Hospital Pharmacy." *Hospitals,* 17(January):58-61.

98. Fuqua, R.F. (1943). "War Requires Use of Few Drug Substitutes in the Carefully Managed Hospital Pharmacy." *Hospitals,* 17(November):73-76.

Chapter 6

1. Anonymous (1898). "Committee on the Status of Pharmacists in the U.S. Army, Navy and Marine Hospital Service." *Proceedings of the APhA,* 46:71-89.

2. "Reorganization of the Medical Dept. 1777, April 7, 1777." In Duncan, L.C. (1931), *Medical Men in the American Revolution 1775-1783.* Carlisle Barracks, PA: Medical Field Service School, p. 194.

3. Anonymous (1894). Proceedings of the APhA;42:vi.

4. Anonymous (1896). Proceedings of the APhA;44-63.

5. Anonymous (1903). Proceedings of the APhA;51:111.

6. Payne, G.F. (1912). "Reasons for Promoting the Status of the Hospital Corps of the United States Army." *Journal of the American Pharmaceutical Association,* 1:95-99.

7. Anonymous (1914). "Report of the Committee on Status of Pharmacists in the Government Service." *Journal of the American Pharmaceutical Association,* 3:1270.

8. Mayo, C. (1915). "President Mayo's Address." *Journal of the American Pharmaceutical Association,* 4:1017-1029.

9. Anonymous (1915). "Report of the Committee on Status of Pharmacists in the Government Service." *Journal of the American Pharmaceutical Association,* 4:1054-1055.

10. Anonymous (1916). "Report of the Committee on Status of Pharmacists in the Government Service." *Journal of the American Pharmaceutical Association,* 5:1037-1038

11. England, J.W. (1917). "Correspondence: Justice to the Pharmacist." *Journal of the American Medical Association,* 68(June 16):1864-1865.

12. Anonymous (1917). "Current Comment: Justice to the Pharmacist." *Journal of the American Medical Association,* 68(June 16):1822.

13. Anonymous (1917). "Report of the Committee on National Defense." *Journal of the American Pharmaceutical Association,* 6:1009-1011.

14. Anonymous (1917). *Journal of the American Pharmaceutical Association,* 6:1004-1008.

15. Stewart, F. E. (1918). "Pharmacology and the Recognition of Professional Pharmacy by the United States Government." *Journal of the American Pharmaceutical Association,* 7:436-442.

16. England, J.W. (1918). "Pharmacy Is an 'Essential Specialty of Army Medical Practice.'" *Journal of the American Pharmaceutical Association,* 7:756-758.

17. Anonymous (1918). "Report of the Committee on the Status of Pharmacists in the Government Service." *Journal of the American Pharmaceutical Association,* 7:815.

18. Ibid., p. 816.

19. Shepardson, F.W. (1918). "The Administration of Pharmacy Problems in Illinois." *Journal of the American Pharmaceutical Association,* 7:1076-1085.

20. Hilton, S.L. (1918). "Supplementary Remarks." *Journal of the American Pharmaceutical Association,* 7:816.

21. House of Representatives Committee on Military Affairs, 65th Congress, second session. Hearings on HR 5531, "To Increase the Efficiency of the Medical Department of the United states Army, to Provide a Pharmaceutical Corps in that department, and to Improve the Status and Efficiency of the Pharmacists in the Army." March 19, 1918, p. 39.

22. Hilton, S. L. (1919). "Report of the Committee on Status of Pharmacists in the Government Service." *Journal of the American Pharmaceutical Association,* 8:1088-1089.

23. Anonymous (1927). "Commissions for Pharmacists in the Reserve Army." *Journal of the American Pharmaceutical Association,* 16:1024-1027.

24. Cook, E.F. (1922). "Report on the Status of Pharmacists in the Army and Navy." *Journal of the American Pharmaceutical Association,* 11:54-57.

25. Ibid., pp. 763-765.

26. Cook, E.F. (1924). "Report on the Status of Pharmacists in the Army and Navy." *Journal of the American Pharmaceutical Association,* 13:262-263.

27. Ibid., pp. 958-959.

28. Cook, E.F. (1928). "Report of the Committee on Pharmacists in Government Service." *Journal of the American Pharmaceutical Association,* 17:1037-1044.

29. House of Representatives Committee on Military Affairs, 70th Congress, second session. Hearings on HR 16278, "A Bill to Amend the National Defense Act by Providing for a Pharmacy Corps in the Medical Department, United States Army," February 20, 1929, 46 pp.

30. Winnie, A.L.I. (1929). "Report of Committee on Pharmacy Corps in the U.S. Army." *Journal of the American Pharmaceutical Association,* 18:1074-1076.

31. Swain, R.L. (1929). "Irregular Legislative Schemes." *Journal of the American Pharmaceutical Association,* 18:1103-1105.

32. Swain, R.L. (1930). "Report of Committee on Pharmacy Corps in the United States Army." *Journal of the American Pharmaceutical Association,* 19:651-652.

33. Anonymous (1930). "A Fatal Error in Dispensing." *Journal of the American Pharmaceutical Association,* 19:910-915.

34. Swain, R.L. (1930). "The Unjustifiable Army System of Dispensing." *Journal of the American Pharmaceutical Association,* 19:808-809.

35. Swain, R.L. (1931). "Report of the Committee on Pharmacy Corps." *Journal of the American Pharmaceutical Association,* 20:977-979.

36. Swain, R.L. (1934). "Report of the Committee on Pharmacy Corps." *Journal of the American Pharmaceutical Association,* 23:632-634.

37. Kendig, E.H. (1935). "Report of the Committee on the Establishment of a Pharmaceutical Corps in the United States Army, 1935." *Journal of the American Pharmaceutical Association,* 24:914-918.

38. Buerki, R.A. (1999). "In Search of Excellence: The First Century of the American Association of Colleges of Pharmacy." *American Journal of Pharmaceutical Education,* 63(fall supplement):55.

39. Kendig, E.H. (1935). "Report of the Committee," p. 918.

40. Ginn, R.V.N. (1997). *The History of the U.S. Army Medical Service Corps.* Washington, DC: Office of the Surgeon General and Center of Military History, United States Army, p. 101.

41. Kendig, E.H. (1937). "Report of the Committee on the Status of Pharmacists in the Government Service." *Journal of the American Pharmaceutical Association,* 26:1050-1051.

42. Kendig, E.H. (1940). "Report of the Committee on the Status of Pharmacists in the Government Service." *Journal of the American Pharmaceutical Association,* Scientific Edition, 29:375-376.

43. Evans, C.H. (1941). "Presidential Address." *Journal of the American Pharmaceutical Association,* Scientific Edition, 30:462.

44. Anonymous (1941). "Committee on Resolutions." *Journal of the American Pharmaceutical Association,* Scientific Edition, 30:547-548.

45. Kendig, E.H. (1942). "Report of the Committee on the Status of Pharmacists in the Government Service." *Journal of the American Pharmaceutical Association,* Scientific Edition, 31:393-399.

46. House of Representatives Committee on Military Affairs, 77th Congress, second session. Hearings on HR 7432, "A Bill to Amend the National Defense Act by Providing for a Pharmacy Corps in the Medical Department, United States Army." November 17, 1942, p. 1.

47. Ibid., p. 8.

48. Ibid., pp. 17-18.

49. Ibid., p. 29.

50. Ibid., p. 30.

51. Ibid., p. 30.

52. Ibid., p. 57.

53. Ibid., p. 68.

54. Ibid., p. 69.

55. Senate Committee on Military Affairs (1943). 78th Congress, first session. Hearings on HR 997, "A Bill to Amend Certain Provisions of the National Defense Act of June 3, 1916, as Amended, Relating to the Medical Department of the Regular Army." June 29, 1943, p. 4.

56. Ibid., p. 9.

57. Ibid., p. 15.

58. Ibid., p. 19.

59. Ibid., p. 24.

60. Ibid., p. 31.

61. Ibid., p. 35.

62. Ibid., p. 39.

63. Kendig, H.E. (1943). "Report of the Committee on the Status of Pharmacists in the Government Service." *Journal of the American Pharmaceutical Association,* Scientific Edition, 32:360-365.

64. Ibid., p. 365.

65. Einbeck, A.H. (1944). "Report of the Committee on the Status of Pharmacists in the Government Services." *Journal of the American Pharmaceutical Association,* Scientific Edition, 33:486.

66. Ibid., p. 487.

67. Ibid.

68. Kendig, H.E. (1994). "Pharmacy and the National Welfare." In Griffenhagen, G.B., Blockstein, W. L., and Krigstein, D. J. (Eds.), *The Remington Lectures: A Century in American Pharmacy.* Washington, DC: American Pharmaceutical Association, pp. 128-136.

Chapter 7

1. House of Representatives Committee on Military Affairs, 77th Congress, second session. Hearings on HR 7432, "A Bill to Amend the National Defense Act by Providing for a Pharmacy Corps in the Medical Department, United States Army." November 17, 1942, p. 1.

2. Duncan, L.C. (1931). *Medical Men in the American Revolution 1775-1783.* Carlisle Barracks, PA: Medical Field Service School, p. 194.

3. Crowley, F.E. (1941). "Pharmacy at an Army Post." *American Professional Pharmacist,* 7:448-450, 462.

4. Armfield, B.B. (1963). *Medical Department United States Army in World War II: Organization and Administration in World War II.* Washington, DC: Department of the Army, p. 313.

5. War Department, U.S. Surgeon General's Office (1943). *Medical Department Supply Catalog.* June 1.

6. House of Representatives Committee on Military Affairs, 77th Congress, second session. Hearings on HR 7432, "A Bill to Amend the National Defense Act by Providing for a Pharmacy Corps in the Medical Department, United States Army." November 17, 1942, p. 8.

7. Kirshner, M. Memories Project Files.

8. Wiltse, C.M. (1968). *Medical Supply in World War II.* Washington, DC: Office of the Surgeon General, p. 74.

9. Armfield, B.B. (1963). *Medical Department United States Army in World War II: Organization and Administration in World War II.* Washington, DC: Department of the Army, p. 56.

10. Noh, J.G. Memories Project Files.

11. Crowley, "Pharmacy at an Army Post."

12. Goldblum, H.H. (1944). "The G.I. Pharmacist." *New Jersey Journal of Pharmacy,* (August-December):2-4.

13. Anonymous (1943). "Old North State." *Southeastern Drug Journal,* 18(December):43, 66.

14. American Pharmaceutical Association (1942). "The Army's Need for Pharmacists." Bulletin No.10-1941-1942. February 3.

15. Gibson, M.R. Memories Project Files.

16. Wisconsin State Board of Pharmacy (1945). Kremers Files, American Institute of the History of Pharmacy Wisconsin series 2636.

17. Mishler, J.W. Jr. Memories Project Files.

18. Berman, A. Memories Project Files.

19. Robinson, C.W. Memories Project Files.

20. Atkins, R.M. Memories Project Files.

21. Fay, J.T. (1999). "Everybody Loved Raymond." *HealthCare Distributor,* (December):8.

22. Griffin, T.E. Memories Project Files.

23. Ginn, R.V.N. (1997). *The History of the U.S. Army Medical Service Corps.* Washington, DC: Center of Military History, U.S. Army, p. 101.

24. Smith, G.K. (1940). "Training Army Pharmacy Technicians." *Journal of the American Pharmaceutical Association,* Practical Pharmacy Edition, 1:296-298.

25. Rubin, I. (1942). "How the Army Makes Pharmacy Technicians Out of Soldiers." *American Druggist,* 105(March):3636-3639.

26. Anonymous (1943). "Professional Notes" *American Society of Hospital Pharmacists Bulletin,* (June):5

27. Smith, G.K. (1940). "Training Army Pharmacy Technicians," pp. 296-298.

28. Rubin, I. (1942). "How the Army Makes Pharmacy Technicians," pp. 36-39.

29. Schwartz, A.T. (1940). "Pharmacy in the U.S. Navy." *Journal of the American Pharmaceutical Association,* Practical Pharmacy Edition, 1:299-301.

30. Younken, H.W. Jr. (1944). "Pharmacy in the Navy." *American Journal of Pharmaceutical Education,* 8:350-357.

31. Briggs, W.P. (1942). "Pharmacy and the Hospital Corps of the U.S. Navy." *Journal of the American Pharmaceutical Association,* Practical Pharmacy Edition, 3:314-320.

32. Higby, W.J. Memories Project Files.

33. Ferguson, D.L. Memories Project Files.

34. Dennis, E.G. (1944). "Pharmacy and the Navy Pharmacist." *Hospital Corps Quarterly,* 17(July):103-108.

35. Colabella, N. (1944). "U.S. Naval Dispensary, Navy Department." *Hospital Corps Quarterly,* 17(July):1-7.

36. Dennis, "Pharmacy and the Navy Pharmacist."

37. Ellinger, J.L. Memories Project Files.

38. Dennis, "Pharmacy and the Navy Pharmacist."

39. Lipes, W.B. (1946). "To Whom It May Concern: Re: Malvin Seibert Aaronson." December 26. Memories Project Files.

40. Bureau of Medicine and Surgery (1942). "Catalog of Hospital Corps Schools and Courses 1942." *Hospital Corps Quarterly,* 16(January):27, 62.

41. Schwartz, "Pharmacy in the U.S. Navy."

42. Anonymous (1944). "A Compendium of Pharmaceuticals." *Hospital Corps Quarterly,* 17(July):50-66.

43. Mullan, F. (1989). *Plagues and Politics: The Story of the United States Public Health Service.* New York: Basic Books, p. 118.

44. Williams, R.C. (1951). *The United States Public Health Service 1798-1950.* Washington, DC: Commissioned Officers Association of the United States Public Health Service, p. 48.

45. Ibid,. pp. 662, 747.

46. Accessed online January 20, 2003. "US Merchant Ships Sunk or Damaged in World War II." <http://www.usmm.org/shipsunkdamaged.html>.

47. Wheeler, M. (1943). "Hospital Corpsmen of the Merchant Marine." *Hospital Corps Quarterly,* 16:106-111.

48. Anonymous (1943). "Pharmacist Training." *The Military Surgeon,* 42:570.

49. Jenkins, E.C. (1944). "Diagnosis and Treatment Aboard Shop by Pharmacist Mates" [lecture]. In *Post Graduate Studies for Pharmacist Mates of the Coast Guard and Maritime Services.* Boston, MA: U.S. Marine Hospital.

50. Wheeler, "Hospital Corpsmen of the Merchant Marine."

51. Archambault, G.F. (1944). "Compounding, Storing and Dispensing of Medicines for the Coast Guard and Merchant Marine Pharmacist Mates. Revised May 17, 1944." Memories Project Files.

52. War Shipping Administration (1944). Operations Regulation No. 67 Stores and Equipment: Standard List of Medical Supplies (Revised) March 13.

53. Ballard, C.W. (1954). *A History of the College of Pharmacy, Columbia University.* New York: Columbia University Press, pp. 47-49.

54. Ibid., p. 49.

55. Brodsky, A. Memories Project Files.

56. Clayton, M.W. Memories Project Files.

57. Curran, F.F. (Ed.) (1995). *Keeping in Touch: Letters from Alumni and Students to the Philadelphia College of Pharmacy & Science During World War II.* Philadelphia: Philadelphia College of Pharmacy & Science, p. 195.

58. Rising, L.W. (1945). "Pharmacists of Seattle Staff Coast Guard Sick Bay." *Pacific Drug Review,* 57(September):58-60.

59. American Council on Education (1942). "Women in the Armed Services." Bulletin 42. December 28.

60. Klein, H.G. (1943). "Meet the Waves' Pharmacist Mates." *Pacific Drug Review,* (May):26-27.

61. Anonymous (1945). "Pharmacists in the WAVES." *American Druggist,* 112(November):96-97, 224, 228.

62. Anonymous (1943). *Arkansas Druggist,* 5(February):6.

63. American Pharmaceutical Association (1944). Bulletin #19-1943-1944. June 13.

64. Henderson M.L. (2002). *American Women Pharmacists: Contributions to the Profession.* Binghamton, NY: Pharmaceutical Products Press, p. 75.

65. Baker, C.A. Memories Project Files.

66. Worthen, D.B. (2002). "Paul Stanley Frament '39—An American Hero." *PostScript,* 13(1):2-3.

Chapter 8

1. Amendment to the Selective Training and Service Act of 1940 Public Law 360 *U.S. Statutes at Large* 77ᵗʰ Congress 1st session, Volume 55 Public Laws. December 20, 1941, pp. 844-846.

2. Elsener, A.L. Memories Project Files.

3. War Department (1945). "Statement by the Secretary of War on War Department Demobilization Plan." Press release May 10, 1945. In Sparrow, J.C. (1951), *History of Personnel Demobilization in the United States Army.* Washington, DC: Office of the Chief of Military History, Department of the Army, pp. 466-472.

4. War Department Chief of Staff Transition from the Point System to a Length-of-Service Policy October 31, 1945. In Sparrow, JC *History of Personnel Demobilization in the United States Army* Office of the Chief of Military History, Department of the Army, 1951 pp. 487-489.

5. Barrett, L.B. (1945). "Some Suggestions for Limitation on Enrollments in Colleges of Pharmacy." *American Journal of Pharmaceutical Education,* 9:234-239.

6. Gilson, C.F. (1945). "A Retail Pharmacist Looks at Postwar Pharmacy." *NARD Journal,* (November 19):2015, 2060, 2062.

7. Posthumous Registration as Pharmacist Wisconsin Board series 2636, 1943/44 Kremers Files, American Institute of the History of Pharmacy.

8. Anonymous (1945). "Now What? From Washington." *American Druggist,* (September):6.

9. Schwartau, N.W. Memories Project Files.

10. Anonymous (1945). "Veterans Must Be Rehired." *NARD Journal,* 20(December):2150.

11. Deery, J.J. (1945). "Rhode Island." *The Apothecary,* (March):48.

12. McAllister, H.C. (1945). "Board of Pharmacy News." *The Carolina Journal of Pharmacy,* 26:403, 405.

13. Edw. N. Hayes (1946, 1949). *The Hayes Druggist Directory.* Detroit: Edw. N. Hayes.

14. State Board of Vocational and Adult Education (1945). *Suggested Outline for Veterans Training in Pharmacy.* Madison, WI: State Board of Vocational and Adult Education.

15. Niemeyer, G., Berman, A., and Francke, D.E. (1952). "Ten Years of the American Society of Hospital Pharmacists, 1942-1952." *Bulletin of the ASHP,* 9:301-317.

16. Fischelis, R.P. and Fiero, G. (1943). "The Civilian Requirements for Pharmacists." *NARD Journal,* 65(October 4):1570, 1572, 1574.

17. Anonymous (1944). "The Supply of Pharmacists." *Bulletin of the ASHP,* 10(August):8.

18. Burlage, H.M. (1945). "The G.I. and Hospital Pharmacy." *The Modern Hospital,* 65(5):102, 104.

19. Anonymous (1948). "Hospital Pharmacy and the Pharmaceutical Survey." *American Professional Pharmacist,* 14:636, 638, 640-643.

20. Olson, K.W. (1974). *The G.I. Bill, the Veterans, and the Colleges.* Lexington: University Press of Kentucky, pp. 15-17.

21. Hines, F.T. (1945). "The Soldiers' Bill of Rights." *Military Surgeon,* 96:11-17.

22. White, A.L. (1945). "Pharmacy and the Returning Veteran." *Proceedings of the Annual Meeting of District 7 of the NABP and the AACP,* (April 6-7):17-21.

23. Hines, "The Soldiers' Bill of Rights."

24. White, "Pharmacy and the Returning Veteran."

25. Office of the Division Commander, Headquarters 31st Infantry Division. General Orders #119 August 25, 1945.

26. Office of the Division Commander, Headquarters 31st Infantry Division. General Orders #118 August 25, 1945.

27. Brittingham, F.W. Memories Project Files.

28. Bennett M.J. (1996). *When Dreams Came True: The GI Bill and the Making of Modern America.* Washington DC: Brassey's, pp. 237-245.

29. Hardwick, M.J. Memories Project Files.

30. Rudd, W.F. (1945). "Too Many Pharmacy Students!!!" *The Virginia Pharmacist,* 29(December):165-166.

31. Anonymous (1945). "Too Many Students?" *The Carolina Journal of Pharmacy,* 27(January):1.

32. Anonymous (1945). "Special Bulletin on Post War Training for the Scientific Professions." *American Journal of Pharmaceutical Education,* 9:460-462.

33. To the Deans of the Colleges American Association of Colleges of Pharmacy April 17, 1946. American Institute of History of Pharmacy Collection housed at the Wisconsin Historical Society, Madison, Wisconsin, Mms 293, Box 36, f 4.

34. Benson, G. Memories Project Files.

35. Anonymous (1946). "15,564 Students Enrolled in 67 Pharmacy Colleges." *Journal of the American Pharmaceutical Association,* Practical Pharmacy Edition, 7:562.

36. Anonymous (1948). "Disabled Veterans Study Pharmacy." *The Merck Report,* (January):3.

37. Crossen, G.E. (1944). "Will Pharmacy Close the Door on the '90 Day Wonders?'" *American Druggist,* July:64-65.

38. Report of the Special Joint Committee on Relations of Boards and Colleges of Pharmacy, as Provided in the Joint Resolutions Adopted by the American Association of Colleges of Pharmacy and the National Association of Boards of Pharmacy. September 1944. American Institute of History of Pharmacy Collection housed at the Wisconsin Historical Society, Madison, Wisconsin, Mms 619, Box 43 f 14.

39. American Council on Pharmaceutical Education Report of the Committee on College Credit for Military Experience May 10, 1944. American Institute of History of Pharmacy Collection housed at the Wisconsin Historical Society, Madison, Wisconsin, Mms 619, Box 43 f 14.

40. Fischelis, R.P. (1945). "Give the Veteran His Due." *Journal of the American Pharmaceutical Association,* Practical Pharmacy Edition, 6:138-139.

41. Mullins, J. Memories Project Files.

42. United States Civil Service Commission (1945). "The Federal Government Needs Pharmacists for War Service Appointments." Announcement 404 (Assembled) October 24.

43. American Pharmaceutical Association (1945). "Civil Service Requirements for Pharmacists." Bulletin No. 22-1944-1945. November 5.

44. Mitchell, H.B. (1945). Letter to R.P. Fischelis, November 8. American Institute of History of Pharmacy Collection housed at the Wisconsin Historical Society, Madison, Wisconsin, Mms 619.

45. Fischelis, R.P. (1945). Letter to H.B. Mitchell, November 30. American Institute of History of Pharmacy Collection housed at the Wisconsin Historical Society, Madison, Wisconsin, Mms 619.

46. American Pharmaceutical Association (1946). "Pharmacy in the Veterans Administration and the Civil Service." Bulletin No. 1, 1946. January 9.

47. Mitchell, H.B. (1946). Letter to R.P. Fischelis, January 11. American Institute of History of Pharmacy Collection housed at the Wisconsin Historical Society, Madison, Wisconsin, Mms 619.

48. Briggs, W.P. (1948). ". . . in the Veterans Administration." *Journal of the American Pharmaceutical Association,* Practical Pharmacy Edition, 9:42-47.

49. Einbeck, A.H. (1945). "Army Must Be Made to Respect the Pharmacy Corps Act." *NARD Journal,* (May 21):837-838.

50. Frates, G.H. (1946). "Brass Hats Give Pharmacy Corps the Brush Off." *NARD Journal,* (March 4):452, 454.

51. Anonymous (1946). "Surgeon General Confers With Committee." *Journal of the American Pharmaceutical Association,* Practical Pharmacy Edition, 7:155-156.

52. Ginn, R.V.N. (1997). The History of the U.S. Army Medical Service Corps Office of the Surgeon General and the Center of Military History. Washington, DC: U.S. Army, p. 201.

53. Einbeck, A.H. (1956). "The History of the Pharmacy Corps." February 29. Manuscript in the Office of the Historian of the Surgeon General of the Army Ginn files, box 4.

54. Ibid.

55. Einbeck, A.H. (1947). "Pharmacy in the Army and Navy." *The Merck Report,* (January):22-226.

56. Ginn, *The History of the U.S. Army Medical Service Corps,* p. 477.

57. Einbeck, "The History of the Pharmacy Corps."

58. Einbeck, "Pharmacy in the Army and Navy."

59. Terkel, S. (1984). *"The Good War."* New York: Ballantine Books.

60. Perrett, G. (1984). *Days of Sadness, Years of Triumph: The American People, 1939-1945.* Madison: University of Wisconsin Press, pp. 441-442.

61. Ibid., pp. 442-443.

Index

Page numbers followed by the letter "f" indicate figures; those folowed by the letter "t" indicate tables.